DUTCH CLASSICS IN HISTORY OF SCIENCE

Published under supervision of the
Netherlands Society
for the History of Medicine, Mathematics and Exact Sciences

XVIII

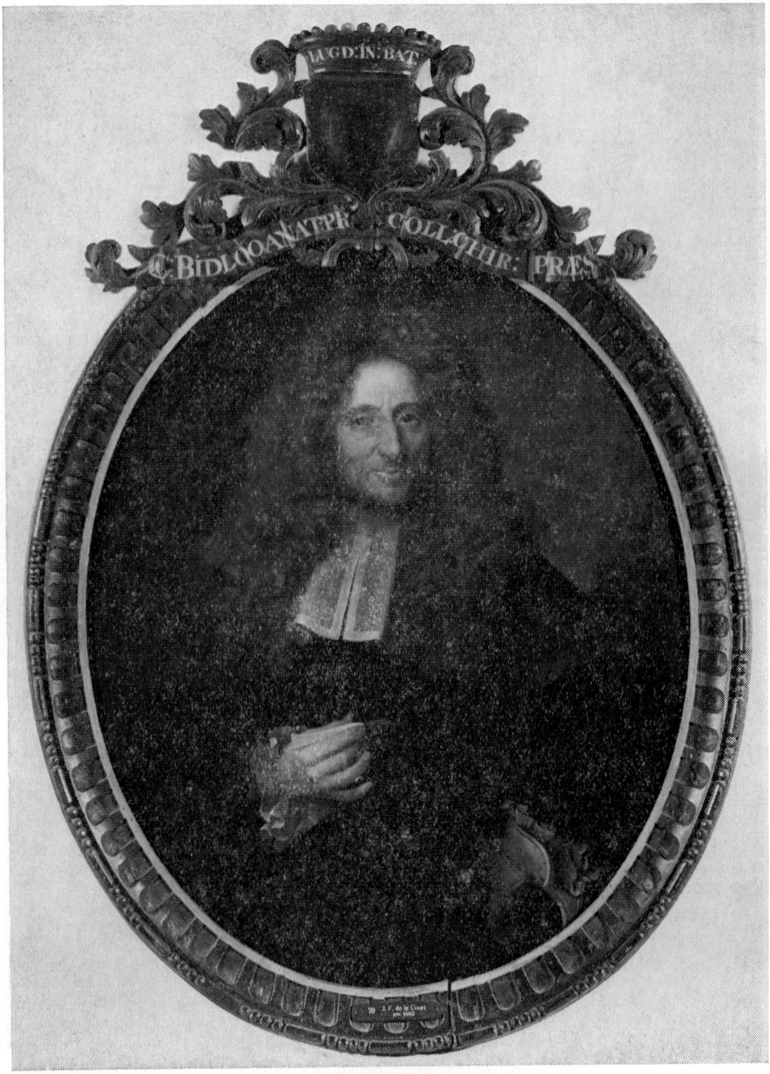
LUGD: IN: BAT
C. BIDLOO ANAT. PR. COLL. CHIR: PRÆS

LETTER FROM G. BIDLOO

TO

ANTONY VAN LEEUWENHOEK

ABOUT THE ANIMALS WHICH ARE SOMETIMES
FOUND IN THE LIVER OF SHEEP
AND OTHER BEASTS

FACSIMILE
of the first Dutch edition – Delft, 1698

With a new English translation,
an introduction and annotations

by

DR. J. JANSEN

NIEUWKOOP * B. DE GRAAF
MCMLXXII

ISBN 90 6004 294 8

TABLE OF CONTENTS

I. INTRODUCTION

Govard Bidloo (1649–1713), the author of the „Brief van G: Bidloo aan Antony van Leeuwenhoek; VVegens de dieren, welke men zomtyds in de lever der Schaapen en andere beesten vind", had a very chequered career. After serving in the army, he was apprenticed to a surgeon, attended the lessons of the anatomist Frederick Ruysch (1638–1731), and three days after his matriculation at Franeker University received a doctor's degree. He then set up as a physician at Amsterdam, may have enlisted in the army once again, became a lecturer in anatomy at The Hague, gave public lectures in anatomy at Rotterdam, in 1690 was appointed Superintendent General of the medical military corps, and in 1692 in a similar function in the English army. In 1694 he received an appointment as a professor at Leyden University and in 1701 he became personal physician to William III, King of England and Stadtholder of the Dutch Republic. He was also a famous poet and playwright in his day (*vide* Krul, 1890; Vasbinder, 1948; Melles, 1961).

Bidloo gained his greatest fame by his big anatomical atlas, published in 1685, which gave rise to extensive polemics and a frequently distasteful quarrel with Ruysch, one of his numerous avowed enemies. In the letter to Antoni van Leeuwenhoek therefore Bidloo does not neglect to criticize the work of Ruysch.

II. ANALYSIS OF BIDLOO'S LETTER TO ANTONI VAN LEEUWENHOEK

A. GOVARD BIDLOO AND ANTONI VAN LEEUWENHOEK

Although Bidloo had many enemies, he had many friends as well. One of the most famous among the latter was Antoni van Leeuwenhoek (1632–1723). It is evident from the opening lines of Bidloo's letter that he was prompted and inspired to study the morphology and habits of the liver fluke *(Fasciola hepatica)* by personal conversations with and letters from his famous compatriot.

The problems connected with the worm in question, the common liver fluke or *F. hepatica*, also roused the interest of Leeuwenhoek, as appears from the information in his letter 42 [27] of 21 February 1679 to the Secretary of the Royal Society; however, according to the edition of „The Collected Letters of Antoni van Leeuwenhoek" (1941) this letter never reached the Royal Society. If this is true, it did not prevent Bidloo from referring to this letter on p. 15.

Already in Leeuwenhoek's letter 12 [7] of 19 October 1674 to the Secretary of the Royal Society he wrote about the eggs which he found in the bile of some animals and which Dobell (1922) rightly took to be eggs of *F. hepatica* (The Collected Letters of Antoni van Leeuwenhoek, 1939). It does not, however, appear from this letter that Leeuwenhoek suspected a connection between these eggs and the liver fluke, though he did later on, considering the letter presumably addressed to Bidloo which the latter mentions on p. 9. This may be the same letter as that cited by Bidloo on p. 16; it was written on 19 January 1698. For that matter, shortly afterwards, in August 1698, Leeuwenhoek again started to search for the liver flukes, as appears from his letter [122] of 2 January 1700 to the Royal Society (Sevende Vervolg der Brieven, 1702).

B. BIDLOO'S INVESTIGATIONS ON THE LIVER FLUKE

Following a sound scientific practice still applied in our day, Bidloo starts by reviewing the pertinent literature (pp. 2–8). Without aiming at completeness, he cites successively Fabritius, Journal des Sçavans, Kircher, Cornelius Gemma, Miscellanea Curiosa (*vide* p. 27 of this introduction), Redi, and finally Ruysch, whose observations he does not fail to depict as worthless.

This survey is followed by his own investigations and notes about the liver fluke, classified as follows: I. morphology (pp. 8–10), II. localization (pp. 10–13), III. numbers and reproduction (pp. 13–20), and IV. etiology of helminthiases (pp. 20–26). Although the description of the morphology starts with „I", the following three numerals were omitted.

The description of the liver fluke is broadly correct, as are the drawings. All this is given in very great detail; as Foster (1965) rightly observes: „in too much detail, describing both eyes and a heart". The description of the eyes (p. 8) can be accounted for by the fact that Bidloo was convinced all animals are bound to have eyes (Vasbinder, 1948), and further by the similarity to flat-fishes observed by him. It even seems to be fairly indifferent to him whether the animalcules are water worms or small fishes (p. 10). The heart also (p. 8) is bound to be present in any animal. One may wonder whether it was not the ventral sucker which Bidloo took to be and drew as the heart. The vascular system (p. 8) is in reality the digestive tract of the fluke. The „very thin pipes or filaments" lying in between are the ramifications of the testes. The intestines (p. 9), which in reality are the uterus, are assumed by Bidloo to end in an anus on the right side of the body. In his drawings this is not visible and the uterus seems to end correctly in what might be the genital pore. From the text one might conclude that the words „on the right side of the body" refer to the anatomy of fishes, but according to the Latin version of the letter (Bidloo, 1698) it is really the body of the worm that is meant. The „blackish globule" (p. 9) might be the ootype, which for the rest is not shown in the drawing. Bidloo then speaks at length about the spawn or eggs of the flukes (p. 9). The remark of Vasbinder (1948) that the testes are described by Bidloo under the name of „spawn" is not correct. Leeuwenhoek's letter mentioned on this page is probably the letter of 19 January 1698 addressed to Bidloo (*vide* p. 16), since in Leeuwenhoek's letter of 19 October 1674 to the Secretary of the Royal Society the flukes and the eggs were not associated with each other. It is striking that Bidloo rightly suspects the flukes to be hermaphrodites (p. 9).

Dispersed among the description of the morphology are also some stray notes on the flukes. Obviously Bidloo only came across chronic infections caused by the liver fluke, for he states that the hosts do not show any clinical symptoms and illness (p. 7), although Leeuwenhoek in his letter of 1679 addressed to the Secretary of the Royal Society mentions that he has found flukes in unhealthy sheep. It should, however, be borne in mind that the connection between the unhealthiness of sheep and the occurrence of liver flukes was not established conclusively until much later. It is indeed astonishing that Bidloo, who was always on the look-out for a connection between the occurrence of worms and the origin of diseases *(vide infra)*, does not comment any further on the observations here referred to. Again the fact that Bidloo never found flukes in the parenchyma of the liver or haemorrhages in the liver (top of p. 12), but did find defects in the bile ducts, goes to prove that he saw only chronic infections. On p. 7 he mentions the influence of temperature and humidity on the flukes as well as their way of locomotion. It is perhaps the same letter of Leeuwenhoek as that mentioned on p. 9 which is cited once more on p. 10, where Bidloo confirms Leeuwenhoek's observation that when many young flukes are found, at the same time many eggs of worms are present. The idea suggested by these observations was that this tended to prove that flukes were produced from eggs in the bile ducts. From the sequel it will become clear that this idea and the resultant conclusions, though understandable, are incorrect.

In discussing the theme of the localization of the flukes Bidloo asserts that they occur only in the system of the bile ducts (pp. 11, 12, 17, 18). The reason why no flukes were found in the parenchyma of the liver has already been given above. Unfortunately Bidloo fails to mention the observation of Faber (1670), who also stated already that the flukes inhabited only the bile ducts, not the blood vessels. A few notes on pathology are also to be found on pp. 11, 12, and 19.

The pages 12 and 15–17 derive their interest from the speculations of Bidloo, Leeuwenhoek, and Redi on the life cycle of the liver fluke. They are found to hold the following – different – views. Redi thinks that the flukes develop in the gall-bladder, after which the young flukes bore and bite through the wall of the main bile duct and get into the veins, not the arteries, of the liver, where they multiply, after which they enter the tissue of the liver through the wall of the blood vessel. Leeuwenhoek (1679) merely mentions that the flukes occur in the blood vessels of the liver. From Bidloo's description in his letter it appears that Leeuwenhoek thought at the time that the flukes, after being swallowed by the host, got through the wall of the stomach and the intestines into the abdomen and migrated thence to the blood vessels of the liver, where they reproduced. Bidloo on the contrary believes that the eggs enter the bile ducts along with the chyle from the intestines via the blood, probably through the portal vein.

It is now known that the eggs cannot develop until they have dropped on the earth along with the faeces via the bile ducts and the digestive tract. The larva leaving the egg, miracidium, infects the snail *Limnaea truncatula* (Bidloo would have boggled at the spelling *Lymnaea!*) and there reproduces via sporocyst and rediae to produce cercariae. The cercariae leaving the snail encyst themselves, mainly on the vegetation, and are then called metacercariae. If the latter are swallowed by the host, the young fluke is liberated from the cyst in the small intestine, bores its way through the wall of the intestine, and via the abdomen reaches the liver. It bores through the capsule of the liver and, after migrating through the tissue of the liver, after a few weeks it reaches the system of the bile ducts.

Redi therefore had some suspicion of the migration through the tissue of the liver and Leeuwenhoek of the migration via the wall of the intestine and the abdomen, while Bidloo remains vague about the migration and merely states clearly that the flukes are to be found only in the bile ducts. Leeuwenhoek later (1700) unfortunately changed his mind. He then asserted that the flukes migrated to the gall-bladder via the ductus choledochus. He did agree at that time that they were not to be found in the blood vessels.

However, all speculations were bound to be erroneous at that time and the research could not but get stuck, because the notion of the alternation of generations, discovered by Steenstrup (1842), was still unknown. It was not until this became known that the complete life cycle of *F. hepatica*, amongst others, could be found (Thomas, first report, 1881).

Subsequently, on the pages 13–20, the numbers of the flukes and their reproduction are discussed. To some extent this part was already commented on above in connection with the migration in the liver. On p. 13 the hosts are mentioned, and it is remarkable that no reference is made here to intra-uterine infections, which were described by Fromann (1675–1676) in a publication actually mentioned by Bidloo (p. 4). As to the occurrence of the flukes in sheep, Bidloo refers to a conversation with or a letter of Leeuwenhoek. In actual fact, no mention is made of this in Leeuwenhoek's letter of 21 February 1679 to the Secretary of the Royal Society.

The statements about man as a host (p. 13) unfortunately have not found their way correctly into the parasitological literature. *F. hepatica* does indeed occur in man, but distinguished parasitologists such as Pallas (1760), Rudolphi (1809), Diesing (1850), Pagenstecher (1879–1893), and Skrjabin (1948) wrongly refer to Bidloo's letter when mentioning man as a host of *F. hepatica*. Reinhard (1957) expresses himself somewhat more cautiously and says that Bidloo saw „similar worms" *(i.e.* similar to *F. hepatica)* in man. These statements ignore the fact that Bidloo says precisely that he is not sure of his ground and that further research is required.

After this part the view that liver flukes might be produced by spontanious generation is refuted in florid language, according to Over (1967) for the first time with respect to *F. hepatica*, and this ends in the rejection of the views of Ruysch, while the thesis of Steenevelt is cited with approval. Afterwards Steenevelt (1700–1701) dedicated the summary of his thesis to Bidloo.

On p. 16 Bidloo accounts correctly for the origin of hydrops ascites, in connection with another incorrect description of the matter by Leeuwenhoek in a letter of 19 January 1698 to Bidloo.

Finally, on pp. 19 and 20, Bidloo criticizes the curious choice of medicaments on the basis of their taste.

C. BIDLOO ON THE ETIOLOGY OF DISEASES

The fourth theme (pp. 20–26) is a discussion meant to show that worms and other small living creatures can be the cause of diseases.

On p. 20 we come across a remark – placed between brackets indeed – which reveals one of the principal motives for Bidloo's investigations: „for ultimately our observations in and about other animals and substances ought to benefit man". This sentence is completed in an excellent way by the remark on p. 34: „. . . I have done this only for the advantage of the medical art and as an incentive to zealous investigators . . ."

To prove that even in man diseases may be caused by worms and other small living creatures, Bidloo enumerates a series of cases from the literature. Only in those instances where a word or term called for an explanation has this been given in the English translation of Bidloo's letter.

D. BIDLOO'S DISCUSSION

The remainder of the letter consists of a general discussion, in which Bidloo seizes the opportunity to set forth once more certain personal views or to expose evil medical practices. To start with, he expounds what value is to be attached to research (pp. 26–29), while he sneers at physicians, the drawing of conclusions from a small number of observations, reliance on stories of others and the Roman Catholic Church, upon which he concludes that the only research that has any value is that which is based on personal study and sound reflection. Finally he again derides a particular form of medical practice, *viz.* quackery, for which he makes use of a Zeedeprint or satirical poem of Constantijn Huygens. According to Eijmaal (1891) the explanation of the verse here quoted is as follows: „raetseer" means one who guesses at the complaint, „praetseer" means a loquacious person, and „raeptseer" is a money-grubber.

On p. 31 Bidloo states that much greater exertion is required to understand diseases than to diagnose them correctly, a truth which is still valid today, and he demonstrates (pp. 31–33) that many of the ailments described are the result rather than the cause of a disease.

At the bottom of p. 33 is to be found a remark that sounds rather hypocritical to the present-day reader, *viz.* that Bidloo will not expatiate any further on themes which really have nothing to do with the subject-matter of the letter and would make it needlessly long for a letter. It should be considered that in those days it was not unusual to dwell in detail on side-issues. Meanwhile this gave Bidloo another excellent opportunity for venting his opinion on all sorts of medical matters (*vide* Vasbinder, 1948), because he thinks (p. 34) that the serious reader will not take this in bad part.

III. CONCLUSIONS

From this letter Bidloo emerges as a sound investigator, who bases his conclusions on scientific thinking, but always keeps in mind the usefulness of the research for man.

The research on the liver fluke, *F. hepatica*, is a well-considered and systematically written study. The only critical remark one might make about the plan is that the detailed review of the literature concerning all sorts of instances of worms and other small living creatures infesting man would be largely superfluous according to present-day standards. In view of the qualities of this letter already the opinion of Krul (1890) that science does not owe Bidloo anything must be contradicted.

Although the subject-matter of the letter is the liver fluke, one cannot help thinking that the research was largely prompted by Bidloo's desire to write in detail on some aspects of the medical art.

As to the latter, he pleads in favour of sound research and criticizes quackery, credulity, and superstition. It is especially when exposing wrong opinions and situations that he runs on at great length and in very florid language, while sneering at all sorts of people and practices.

IV. EDITIONS OF BIDLOO'S LETTER TO ANTONI VAN LEEUWENHOEK

1698 Brief van G: Bidloo, aan Antony van Leeuwenhoek; VVegens de dieren, welke men zomtyds in de lever der Schaapen en andere beesten vind. Gedrukt te Delft, by Henrik van Kroonevelt, Boekverkooper. 1698.

1698 Godefridi Bidloo; Observatio, de animalculis, In ovino aliorumque animantium hepate detectis, Ad virum celebrem Antonium van Leeuwenhoek. Lugd. Batav. Apud Jordanum Luchtmans, 1698. (Preceded by an account of four pages.)

1698 Observatio Medico-anatomica, de animalculis, in ovino aliorumque animantium hepate, detegendis; quam Deo propitio, sub Praesidio Viri Excellentissimi ac Experientissimi, D. D. Godefridi Bidloo, Anatom. & Colleg. Chirurg. ejusdem civitatis, Praesidis, Publicè defendendam suscipit, Henricus Snellen, ... Lugduni Batavorum, Apud Abrahamum Elzevier, Academiae Typographum. MDCXCVIII. (Snellen defended the above mentioned Latin paper written by Bidloo. The copy in the British Museum consists of Bidloo's Letter written in Latin with an extra front-page, with the above mentioned text, added.)

1700 Godefridi Bidloo; Observatio de animalculis in ovino aliorumque animantium hepate detectis. Abstract in: Phil. Tr. Roy. Soc. London, s. B., v. 22, pp. 571–572, (1700–1701).

1715 Godefridi Bidloo; Observatio de animalculis in ovino aliorumque animantium hepate detectis, Ad virum celebrem Antonium van Leeuwenhoek. In: Opera omnia anatomico-chirurgica, edita et inedita quorum sequens pagina seriem continet. Lugd. Batav.

1798 Of an animalcule or small living Creature, which is sometimes found in the livers of Sheep and other beasts. (Extract and translation of the „Brief van G: Bidloo," etc. by S. Hoole in: Select Works of A. van Leeuwenhoek. Vol. 1., Part. 2., pp. a-f, London.)

1948 Brief van G. Bidloo aan Antony van Leeuwenhoek; Wegens de dieren, welke men zomtijds in de lever der Schaapen en andere beesten vind. (Extract in: W. Vasbinder; Govard Bidloo en William Cowper. Diss. Utrecht, 1948, pp. 225–227.)

NOTE

The Index-Catalogue of Medical and Veterinary Zoology (U.S. Dept. of Agriculture, Washington) on p. 368 further mentions the following edition: „(1697 a) – Observatio de animalculis in ovino aliorumque animantium hepate detectis. Leidae." It is unlikely that this edition really exists: 1. The bracketing of the date means that the compilers of the Index-Catalogue were unable to verify the reference; 2. The notation „Leidae" for the place of publication instead of „Lugduni Batavorum" militates against the edition; 3. The letter in Dutch bears the date 21 March 1698 on the last page; 4. Prior to the Latin edition of his letter in 1698 Bidloo himself renders an account of the publication in Latin; it may be assumed that Bidloo first wrote, and perhaps even published, his letter in Dutch, since Antoni van Leeuwenhoek had no command of Latin; in fact some words in the Latin edition are yet in Dutch.

V. REFERENCES

Godefridi Bidloo; Observatio, de animalculis, in ovino aliorumque animantium hepate detectis, ad virum celebrem Antonium van Leeuwenhoek. Lugd. Batav. Apud Jordanum Luchtmans, 1698.

Diesing, C. M.; Systema helminthum. Vol. I. Vindobonae, 1850.

Dobell, C.; The discovery of the Coccidia. Parasitology, v. 14, pp. 342–348, (1922).

Joh. Faber; Note in G. J. Sachs' Scholium to Th. Bartholin's Sanguis verminosus. Lipsiae, 1670, obs. 50., p. 147. (After Pagenstecher).

Foster, W. D.; A history of parasitology. Edinburgh and London, 1965.

Joh. Christianus Fromann; De verminoso in ovibus et juvencis reperto hepate. Misc. Acad. Nat. Curios., v. 6–7, pp. 245–252, (1675–1676).

Hoole, S.; Select works of Leeuwenhoek. Vol. I. Part. 2., London, 1798.

C. Huygens' Zede-printen, vermeerderd met de tot dusver onuitgegeven print van „een professor" en van inleiding en aanteekeningen voorzien door H. J. Eijmaal. Groningen, 1891.

Index-Catalogue of Medical and Veterinary Zoology. (U.S. Dept. of Agriculture, Washington), Part. 2., p. 368, (1937).

Krul, R.; Govard Bidloo. Haagsch Jaarboekje voor 1890, v. 2., pp. 49–75, (1890).

Antoni van Leeuwenhoek; Brief, 12 [7], van 19 October 1674 aan H. Oldenburgh. The Collected Letters of Antoni van Leeuwenhoek. Amsterdam, Vol. I., pp. 168–187, (1939).

Antoni van Leeuwenhoek; Brief, 42 [27], van 21 Februari 1679 aan N. Grew. The Collected Letters of Antoni van Leeuwenhoek. Amsterdam, Vol. II., pp. 408–423, (1941).

Antoni van Leeuwenhoek; Brief, [122], van 2 Januari 1700 aan Hans Sloane, secretaris van de Royal Society. Sevende Vervolg der Brieven. Delft, By Henrik van Krooneveld, pp. 152–166, (1702).

Antoni van Leeuwenhoek; Brief, [152], van 3 November 1703 aan de leden van de Royal Society. Not published. Original Letter in Royal Society, Early Letters, L. 3,54. English translation of a part of it in: Philosophical Transactions Roy. Soc., London, no. 289, v. 24., pp. 1522–1527, (1704).

Melles, J.; Rotterdamse chirurgijns in vroeger eeuwen. Nieuwe Rotterdamse Courant, Wekelijks bijvoegsel, 18 November 1961, no. 46, p. 1.

Over, H. J.; Ecological biogeography of *Lymnaea truncatula* in the Netherlands. Diss. Utrecht, 1967.

Pagenstecher, H. A.; in Pagenstecher, H. A. und Braun, M.; Würmer: Vermes. Bronn's Klassen und Ordnungen des Thier-Reichs. IV Band. Leipzig, 1887–1893.

Petrus Simon Pallas; Dissertatio medica inauguralis de Infestis Viventibus intra Viventia. Lugduni Batavorum, apud Theodorum Haak, 1760.

Reinhard, E. G.; Landmarks of parasitology I. The discovery of the life cycle of the liver fluke. Exp. Parasitol., v. 6, pp. 208–232, (1957).

Rudolphi, C. A.; Entozoorum sive Vermium Intestinalium historia naturalis. Vol. II. P. I., Amstelaedami, 1809.

Skrjabin, K. I.; Trematodes of animals and man. Vol. II. Moscow-Leningrad, 1948. (In Russian).

Christiani à Steenevelt; Dissertatio de ulcere verminoso ad clarissimum virum Godefridum Bidloo. Phil. Tr. Roy. Soc. London, v. 22, pp. 570–571, (1700–1701).

Steenstrup, J. J. S.; Om Fortplantning og Udvikling gjennem vexlende Generationskraekker, en saeregen Form for Opfostringen i de lavere Dyrklasser. Kjøbenhavn, 1842.

Thomas, A. Ph. W.; Report of experiments on the development of the liver-fluke *(Fasciola hepatica)*. J. Roy. Agric., Soc. England, v. 17, pp. 1–29, (1881).

Vasbinder, W.; Govard Bidloo en William Cowper. Diss. Utrecht, 1948.

REMARKS

The references in the Letter are made more accesible by the consultation of the Latin edition of the Letter (1698) and the Index-Catalogue of Medical and Veterinary Zoology. For complete information the reader is referred to reference catalogues like the Index-Catalogue mentioned above.

Additions and explanations have been placed between square brackets.

The numbers of the pages of the original letter have been placed between normal brackets.

Misc. Cur. means: Miscellanea Curiosa, sive Ephemeridum Medico-Physicarum Germanicarum Academiae Naturae Curiosum.

Acta Hafn. means: Acta Regiae Societatis Medicae Havniensis, Havniae.

LETTER FROM G. BIDLOO
TO ANTONY VAN LEEUWENHOEK

About the animals which are sometimes found in the liver of sheep and other beasts.

G. BIDLOO *wishes the famous Mr. ANTONI van* (1)
LEEUWENHOEK may make progress, find pleasure, and earn glory in his diligent examination of animal bodies and other substances.

Dear Sir,

Your courteous letters, kind reception, and pleasant discussions on many interesting things induce me respectfully to present to you the following observa-
tion, on which we recently had a conversation, the (2)
more so because I have become fully convinced of its truth also through your own observations and speculations.

After I had frequently found, now accidentally, now intentionally, in the liver of human beings and beasts various diseases, tumours, stones, substances, and especially in those of sheep a kind of animals the name (worms), description, and representation of which seemed to me not to be in agreement with their constitution, or at least very little, I did my best to investigate this. But as I have always detested the odious habit of disparaging the work of others, I looked up, before saying anything on the subject, what famous, learned, and zealous men might have discovered about this. Amongst them – to avoid searching everywhere and at random – I glanced through the authors of recent times and of our own day, and found that the never sufficiently praised FABRITIUS HILDANUS, in the first Part of his Observationum et curationum chirurgicarum centuriae, page 74, asks: *What is more curious, what is more astonishing than that worms are found in the gall-bladder?* Nevertheless I found this confirmed by the statement and the authority of the reliable Mr. GALENUS WIERUS, in his letter written from Düsseldorf on the 16th of June of the year 1602.

The French (see their journal, under the title of *Journal*
(3) *des Sçavans*, published in the year 1668), being engaged in a detailed examination of the duct through which the bile is conveyed to the duct of the gall-bladder, found in the bile ducts of a sheep these so-called worms, and some of them, since at that time there was a general fear in Paris of the Plague and they had perhaps read the treatise by ATH. KIRCHERUS on the Plague, published in the year 1658, wanted to have it considered whether

these animalcules might not be forebodings of that sad disease, while Corn. Gemma speaks of something similar that happened in Holland around the year 1562; he maintains that the frequent diseases and high mortality among the cattle are forebodings of those of men. They compare the form of the animalcule to that of skull cap [*Scutellaria minor*], which grows in the fields, and further describe it as follows: *They are flat, oval, and somewhat pointed towards one end of the edge; the head protrudes a little at the other end, which stands for the stalk of the leaf. They are whitish on the belly; on the back they are covered with many spots and threads of a dark brown colour, which makes them resemble the sole. The head has a snout with a small hole in it, in addition to another which is much larger and is found near the middle towards the bottom.* They add the following illustration and this explanation:

1. Denotes the animalcule lying on its back, 2. lying on its belly, 3. the leaf of the above-mentioned plant as described by Bauhinus.

They do not add anything further except a general (4)
discussion about the uncertainty of the prognoses, predictions, and forebodings of the plague.

What Messrs. Bartholinus, Fabritius, Hauptmannus, Tardinus and others say about these as well as some other animalcules is found collected in the accurate Misc. Cur. in the year 1670 on p. 128 and in 1675, 1676 in the observations of Mr. Fromannus on p. 249

and subsequent pages. At about the same time, to wit in
the year 1671, Mr. FRANCISCUS REDI, known univer-
sally because of his merit, in his Experimenta circa
(5) generationem insectorum, p. 302, also speaks about
these animalcules and depicts their form as follows:
He compares them to a pumpkin seed [Cucurbita pepo] or a small myrtle leaf [Myrthus communis] with a short stalk; and he further says *that they are a milky white and provided with yellowish green ducts; they have a mouth or hole not far from the tail, in the surface of the belly; they are often found not only in the gall-bladder, but also in all the vessels of the liver, except the arteries, of sheep.* Which of all these statements are to be accepted according to my experience, you may see in the sequel.

Finally I found that also Mr. FRED. RUYSCH, on p. 84
of his observations [Dilucidatio valvularum in vasis
lymphaticis et lacteis], makes mention of the aforesaid
animalcules. But how far his description deviates from
the truth and the form of this animalcule (for he says
little about it except this and the place where it was
found by him in the liver of sheep) will become ap-
(6) parent when one compares his description with my
true one; for I trust no one will take this picture to be
that of an animal, as it has nothing bearing any sem-
blance to a living creature, but one will rather take it to
be a glandular tissue or some other substance. Never-
theless he says, referring to letter E. *worms taken out of*

the duct of the gall-bladder and the bile ducts of a sheep.

To arrange my discussion of the said animalcule intelligibly, I will start my remarks and observations first with its body; secondly, the places where it is found; thirdly, their number, birth, and reproduction; and fourthly, I will show that these and other animalcules, living in the liver and other parts of the body, may cause certain diseases and their symptoms.

I. As to the form, contour, and resemblance of these animalcules, which are compared (apart from the aforesaid resemblances) now to the leaf of moneywort
[Lysimachia nummularia], now to a leech, it bears a (7)
great likeness, in miniature, to our fish the sole or the flounder, as can be seen in the first drawing, in which A. designates one of these animalcules, in the size in which they are generally found, on the convex side or the back, B. the same turned upside down and therefore seen from the side of the belly, C. shows one of the young of the animalcule, viewed in the first way, and D. in the second way. Under letters E. and F. the animalcule is drawn with the whole body somewhat magnified, on both sides.

They are seldom seen alive, because the disease cannot be told by outward signs and the beast that suffers from it sometimes appears fat and healthy; and the liver is not examined until after death, while these animalcules also cannot endure cold or the addition of

another fluid. I saw them alive, after having frequently stayed during the slaughtering specially arranged for that purpose, and the last time on the 13th of March in large numbers, as well as at the same time a kind of short, thick worms [not determinable] in the liver of a cat. When they begin to grow cold and thus become motionless, they resume their motion when they are held in a warm hand or when the liver is laid in warm water. Their motion is like that of the above-mentioned fishes, *i.e.* undulating, the sides of the body being rolled round as they progress, and thus the head being first drawn towards the trunk, the body broadened, and then
(8) stretched lengthwise. Their colour is a brownish yellow, the belly is quite flat and much paler than the back. Further their skin is rough, covered with points, and so transparent that the intestines and vessels can be seen through it on either side. Their head (see the magnified drawing under letter G.) has the form of a truncated cone, the mouth projecting upwards and oval when open, almost like that of a carp. The eyes (see as above, under the letters H. and I.), which protrude very much, are surrounded by a cartilaginous ring K., and, as in many flat-fishes, are placed not on either side, but on one side of the head.

The heart is so near to the head, and the intestines again are so close to the heart, that I doubt whether there is anything by which the head is distinguished

from the rest of the body, which yet in most animals is the case. From the heart two vessels spread through the whole body, leaving a wide interstice in the middle of the back, along its length, in the way to be seen under letter L.; between them, under letter M., extend very thin pipes or filaments, in which no fluid can be perceived. In the former vessels I find two kinds of fluid, *viz.* in some, brownish-yellow and sometimes purplish, in others, pale green, both always mucous, but yet flowing (even when the animalcule is dead and is held up by the hind part) towards the heart and away from it
again, when the head is raised, towards the hind part of (9)
the body. Some gentlemen wondered that when the animalcules are alive this flowing to and fro takes place much more slowly (though nevertheless the fluid in them is thinner while they are alive than after their death) than when they are dead; but when they thought of the deferent ducts and the propulsive motion of the heart, the reason and consequently the effect of the argument became plain and evident to them.

The intestines have their exit or navel – that is how, through a bad habit, this opening is called in fishes – on the right side of the body, very shortly beneath the head, so that they are compressed very much. A blackish globule, placed at the beginning of the intestines, I assume to be the liver.

Between this and the intestines I find, in all the

animalcules examined by me, the innumerable quantity of oval particles of which you speak in your letter, and I have found, like you, that hundreds of them when taken together, hardly reaching the size of a coarse grain of sand, have a faint red colour. They appear to me to be the spawn or eggs of these animalcules. But in spite of my diligent efforts I have not yet succeeded in distinguishing the sex of each animalcule with complete certainty; being frequently in doubt, it seems to me to come closest to the truth that they belong to that kind of animals in which both sexes are present, or that so
(10) far I have not got hold of a male. How far the number of females exceeds that of the males in some aquatic animals is found, amongst others, in haddocks. It is not relevant whether these animals should be called water worms or fishes, since the same is also found in animals living on the land, like slugs and others. The smallness of the body also is not to the point, for there are many kinds of water and land animals of the same size and growth. Nay, thousands which are a thousand times smaller and have various forms are seen daily, even in rain-water. I request you to give your comment on the above. I also find, as you saw fit to inform me, that wherever one sees young specimens of these animalcules, many of the above-mentioned oval particles make their appearance in the fluid, being dark-coloured bile, in which they lie, which particles, however small they

are, yet are all found to have one and the same form and to be transparent.

The tail or the lower end, though similar to the whole body, is much tenderer than any of the other exterior parts, breaking at the slightest rough touch.

The only places in which I have so far found these animalcules are the vessels, ducts, and receptacles for the use of the bile, but they are most numerous in the bile ducts, which in that case protrude everywhere beyond measure and in great protuberances, windings,
bends, and little cavities, the diameter of which is often (11)
an inch and a half, in the sites where these animalcules are found heaped together, and those sites are also hard like cartilage. In the small bile ducts they lie lengthwise and sometimes rolled up at least three times, and I believe that it is due to this that many people, being deceived as to their form, have described them as elongated, round worms. And yet, however folded up they may be, still they at once expand and resume their flat form, even after their death, when thrown into warm water; but they also change their colour somewhat (to wit: they become pale).

One seldom sees these animalcules without tumours or ulcers being visible in the liver at the same time. But however many or few, small or big the animalcules were, I never found any alteration in the usual form of the blood-vessels, with any exception, or in the blood therein; even less so did I find the animalcules in the vessels, the nerves perfectly preserving their general course, extension, and constitution. I find the lymphatic vessels throughout the body different from their usual condition, some being excessively expanded, others quite flat, nay, hardly visible, and the abdomen is full of lymph in that case; the glandular tissue of the liver, in its interstices, much distended and inflated, every gland filled and permeated with fluid, separately visible, and as it were separated from its neighbour, even the outer membrane of the liver thicker and harder than usual.

(12) It will be very plausible that these animalcules never inhabit the tissue of the liver or its blood-vessels when it is argued that they must be introduced into them either from the outside – which no one is likely to assert – or through the blood-vessels, bile ducts, or lymphatic vessels.

Firstly, as the arteries are heavily built and further very narrow, even so narrow near their ends in the liver that they can contain none of these animalcules (I here keep silent on the counter-argument to be derived from the motion of the blood and other causes), I conclude with Mr. Redi that it is impossible that they can stay and grow in the arteries, but nevertheless, contrary to his opinion (with all due deference to his great reputation), I consider that they are not present in the other blood-vessels either. For if (as he asserts) they are

brought forth in the gall-bladder and, having crept through it, pierce by biting through the common bile duct and thence again through and into the blood-vessels, one would have to see everywhere blood that has been shed or is flowing out, which I have never yet found. That they should there, after multiplication, again gnaw through the blood-vessels, thus penetrate into the glandular tissue of the liver and make little cavities there, apart from its improbability is also contrary to experience, since the minutest bile ducts, when these animalcules are present therein, even near the thinnest edge of the liver, are so expanded, enlarged, and widened that its glandular tissue is united with the
outer membrane, not the least substance resembling (13)
blood being found in the little cavities.

The number of these animalcules is commonly large, yet it varies and depends on whether they have had more or less time to propagate. Out of one liver I could produce 870 whole specimens besides many that were broken and injured during dissection and extraction; out of another, only 10 or 12. They are found in various kinds of beasts. Hunters on the Veluwe tell me that they have found them in deer, wild boars, and other big and small game. I often saw them in calves and in a young bullock, a few days ago in a heifer, but they were greenish black. It has long been known to many people and to you that they are found in sheep even

from the womb, in lambs one year old and upwards, and even in aged sheep. I often found on and near the liver of human beings worms, but of quite a different form and constitution. Although, now that I have come to know the animalcules in question in more detail, and in particular how they can roll themselves up, I venture to think that I saw them some years ago in a human liver, yet, before affirming this, I will take every opportunity (and I request you to do the same) to discover the truth about this. As to the birth, first cause, substance, and reproduction of these animalcules, which some authors try to attribute to putrefaction,
(14) corruption, lack of salt, intemperate moistness or heat, and other silly ideas, words, and qualities, such as that, once they have been produced from putrid matter, *Multiplicativi sui mediante sive operante facultate foventrice* [read: *Multiplicativa* as in Latin edition; (they are) self-multiplying by means of or rather through a cherishing ability], and other idle talk, I reject it all and I firmly believe that these animalcules, like all *living* or moving things, are produced from their like, *i.e.* from eggs, seed, spawn, briefly a substance similar to them as they arose and of the same constitution. For I consider that the age in which we are living has progressed too much in the knowledge of tangible and visible (let alone other) things, too much in the proper foundation of argumentation, and too much on the road of proper

inquiry for us to occupy ourselves and others any longer with such stuffy and dull old wives' and dribbling children's tales, which on the basis of unenlightened paganism are more in agreement with a fairy tale of an imagined Morpheus or a Lallus at the cradle than with a decent conversation of even moderately intelligent people. I should discuss the above subject at greater length if this matter had not been dealt with in detail a short time ago by Mr. C. VAN STEENEVELD in the Dissertatio de Ulcere Verminoso, in which, refuting the 64th of the observations written by Mr. FR. RUYSCH, he clearly convinces the latter of the aforesaid truth. See the aforesaid treatise, pp. 9–18, where you will find your name honoured and your findings mentioned, to (15)
reinforce the evidence.

I consider that the circumstances under which, as you already wrote to the Royal Society in England in 1679, you think these animalcules and their eggs get into sheep (for other animalcules and their eggs the same will have to be assumed), *viz.* that in rainy summer and autumn periods, coming out of the earth, they are swallowed with the fluid in which they live or into which they get, are very probable (having received information on this from farmers, graziers, and butchers), but (with my apologies to you) I believe by no means that, forcing their way through stomach and intestines, they penetrate from the abdomen into the vessels of the liver, propagate there, and, making openings in the stomach and intestines, are the effective causes that (out of those holes) the large amount of fluid that is sometimes found in the abdomen is poured out and trickles out. For if, now already in the form of animalcules, they get into the stomach and intestines, if they can force their way through them at all, they will no doubt also be able to penetrate through the membranes of the other intestines lying on and near the aforesaid ones, such as the pancreas, kidneys, and spleen, and will be found therein (which I have never yet seen).

Add to this, secondly, that they would then be sufficiently visible everywhere, and must also always be found at least in the stomach or intestines (which again does not happen).

(16) Thirdly, even if they made their way through the aforesaid parts, chyle or a fluid as thin as chyle would have to flow therefrom. Otherwise, if the fluid were thicker, one ought to discover the holes in those intestines. To find out the truth about this, I compressed and searched the stomach and intestines of a sheep that was harassed in the extreme by this complaint, while they were [still] warm, subsequently held them in warm water, filled them with warm water, then again poured warm brandy and finally mercury into the lowermost part, and then agitated them, compressed them again

and again, examined them, and treated them in all ways I could think of, but I could not detect any openings in them at all. That they should crawl out of the duodenum through the common bile duct into the gall-bladder and bile ducts, produce their young there, etc. is too much at variance with the known constitution and operation or use of these parts than that I should have to refute this.

The ideas given by you in your letter of the 19th of January last, as to the drinking of canal water and [its use in the] preparation of food for human beings, *viz.* that many animalcules (I mean: aquatic animalcules and their eggs) may thus get into the human body, please me very much, but I firmly believe that the lymph which is found in the abdomen, as stated above, in human beings and beasts oozes only from burst, broken, or otherwise injured lymphatic vessels, but does not leak from the holes which these animalcules make in the stomach or the intestines. But I understand (17)
at the same time that these animalcules, though not present in the lymphatic vessels themselves, can break and injure the lymphatic vessels and their beginnings in the liver, it being to me an indubitable truth that the semen or the eggs of these as well as other animalcules (for this, see pp. 12 and 13 of the treatise by Mr. STEENEVELD) can get with the chyle into the blood, with the blood into the liver (in particular with respect to these

animalcules), and further only into the bile ducts and organs, stay there, propagate, and thus tear and rupture the adjacent parts.

Firstly, they inhabit neither the blood-vessels in general nor those of the liver in particular, because they have nothing (I except to some extent the portal vein) in and through which they differ essentially from the general blood-vessels. I say: they are not in the blood-vessels, because of their own continuous, proper, and progressive movement as well as that of the blood and the fluids admixed therewith.

Secondly, not in the lymphatic vessels, for the above-mentioned reason: their narrowness and their continuous discharge of fluid from a narrow to a wider place.

Thirdly, not in the nerves, because these are not hollow ducts whose ends open out into the lumen of the bile ducts.

Fourthly, not in and between the membrane enclosing the portal vein and the bile ducts, since this closely fits everywhere without interstices and itself
(18) also has no open ducts continuing in the bile ducts, in which alone these animalcules are found.

Fifthly again, not between and in the places where artery and vein, coming together after indefinite ramification and division from their trunk and further from larger into smaller branches in the form of a small blot, build up the glands. These places also being so small and pre-eminently destined for the transfusion of the blood as well as the secretion of the lymph and for the purpose of nutrition, and further destined for continuous movement, it is not to be understood that they could serve for the reproduction of these animalcules.

Sixthly, even less so in the membrane enveloping the liver, or the umbilical cord, already changed into a ligament, or in the system of sinews and membranes connecting the liver with the diaphragm. I therefore think I may conclude, according to reason and from my experience, that these animalcules can be produced, grow, and multiply their kind again only in the organs, ducts, and receptacles of the bile. As further evidence of this statement may serve the following. Firstly, the thought that the semen, the spawn or eggs of these animalcules, conveyed along with the oily part of the chyle in the beast infested with them by the blood into the bile organs, can be fastened and rest there, the walls of those vessels always being covered with a
mucous and sticky fluid. Add to this that the bile is not, (19)
like the blood, in continuous motion, its efferent duct, after having passed a short distance between the membranes of the intestines, being closed with a circle of muscle fibres, so that it may be now closed, now open, according to requirement.

Secondly, where these animalcules or their eggs are

found, the bile ducts are swollen and hard, and have changed their colour, the animalcules themselves adhering so firmly to the aforesaid thick bile that their bodies, even if removed [out of the ducts], are yet covered therewith on all sides.

Thirdly, the fluid that is squeezed out of their mouth and navel is the same as, only a little thinner than that in which they live and by some components of which they are nourished. But is this to be wondered at? Every animal has its own living site and nutriment, as its constitution requires. Sea-fish die in fresh water, river-fish in salt water, a worm in the air, a bird in the ground, and so on. It is small wonder (I therefore say) that this animalcule, once it has got into the body of another animal, lives, grows, propagates, and is found only in its own living site and on its own nutriment or such as resembles it most, to wit in the organs of the bile and in the bile itself. I therefore deem it quite an ill-founded doctrine that in order to drive worms and other animalcules out of people's bodies one should give them only bitter medicaments, for one always sees the contrary in some diseases caused by worms. Let
(20) toothache be an example: to cure this, by bringing honey, sugar, or some other sweet substance near the decayed teeth one removes worms from them and thus cures the illness.

Now to show that these animalcules as well as

others, present in the liver and other places and parts of bodies, are the cause of some diseases and the symptoms connected therewith, one should know in general that hardly any substances can be mentioned in which animalcules are not sometimes found. Anyone wishing to have some idea of this should read the observation written by Mr. Philippus Schas van Leeuwenheimb [read: Sachs von] and published in the Misc. Cur. under the year 1670, pages 34 and following. But, to put it briefly, one should know in particular, even apart from other creatures, that no such fluid or solid parts in man can be mentioned (for ultimately our observations in and about other animals and substances ought to benefit man) in and about which our constantly searching zeal for the last few years (your example should be praised!) has not discovered living animalcules.

I do not want to assert (because it is contrary to the truth) that one can always demonstrate that in all diseases, itchings, herpes and ring-worm, ulcers, and tumours it is animalcules, and especially those here mentioned, which are the cause, for I know that from some pustules a substance is squeezed which resembles
nothing more than a worm and which is yet nothing (21)
less than a worm. Here follows a summary of cases and places where animalcules, worms, and other creatures have been found in human bodies by men of judgment

and zeal, for if I were to put forward a collection of the nonsense that could be found on the subject, about the strange metamorphosis, reproduction, and biting and piercing force of these animalcules and others, I should make too high demands on time, your knowledge of these things, and my patience.

Worms then have been *found in the head;* see the aforesaid Misc. Cur., first 100, Year 2, Observation 147 and Year 3, Obs. 414; second 100, under Years 9 and 10, Obs. 50.

Forty pin-worms [It is doubtful whether pin-worms were really meant], *expelled* by an old woman *through the nostrils* after she had suffered from severe migraine, are mentioned by P. BORELLUS in his treatise Historiarum et observationum medico-physicarum, both in the epilogue and in Obs. 19 and 39.

A worm was found *on the dura mater*, as reported by FORESTUS in his 9th Letter, Obs. 4, of the first Part [Observationum et curationum medicinalium ac chirurgicarum].

A similar thing is reported by HILDANUS, in the first 100, Obs. 16; and also a worm expelled *through the nose*, as above, Obs. 8 [Observationum et curationum chirurgicarum].

Worms of the eyes are mentioned by PECHLINUS in his 2nd Book, Obs. 35 [Observationes physico-med.].
(22) How they were *expelled from the nose*, we read in

Forestus [l.c.], Book 21, Obs. 26, Part 3. The Misc. Cur., second 100, Year 3, Obs. 99; in Tulp [Observationes medicae], Book 4, Chapter 12; P. Borellus [l.c.], third 100, Obs. 45.

How many times *worms* are found *in the ears* is to be found in the aforesaid Misc. Cur., Years 3 and 4, Obs. 5. In Forestus [l.c.], Book 21, Obs. 26, in Book 12, Obs. 9; Plinus [Plinius, Historiae mundi], Book 20, Chapter 14; J. B. Montanus [De excrementis], Obs. 40.

Toothache worms are mentioned by Pechlinus [l.c.], Book 2, Obs. 36.

A series of cases of *worms of the teeth themselves* are found reported in the aforesaid Misc. Cur., see Year 5, Obs. 192; Years 9 and 10, Obs. 24 and 187. In the Acta Hafn., Part 5, Obs. 108, and Leeuwenhoek [Letter dated September 17, 1683; abstract in Phil. Tr. Roy. Soc. London (159), vol. 14, pp. 568–574 (1684)]. That *worms* are swimming *in the saliva*, is described, besides in the Misc. Cur., Years 9 and 10, Obs. 130, by many others, Hildanus [l.c.] saying in his first Part, Obs. 59, that a great many of them inhabiting *the gums* were the cause of death.

Worms come out of the backbone according to the German records, see [Misc. Cur.], Year 2, Obs. 10 [read: 109]. Petrus Borellus [l.c.] finds them *on the back* and calls them, after the site, *worms of the back:* Part 1, Obs. 89. Not only worms, but *slugs* also are sometimes

ejected from the body by vomiting; see as above, Misc.
(23) Cur., Obs. 85 in the first Part of Year 3. Infinite is the number of observations that are found about *worms vomited out of the stomach*. Thus the Misc. Cur. speak of them in Year 3, Obs. 258, idem, and Year 4, Obs. 38 and 80, in the second Part; Year 4, Obs. 39; Year 6, Obs. 33.

These worms, but white and longer, are discussed by FORESTUS [l.c.], in Book 21, Obs. 26, and also in the same place that an old man had spat out 500, and another 300.

That *cardalgia* is caused *by worms* is asserted by the physicians of Copenhagen, [Acta Hafn.], in Part 5, Obs. 34.

That there are *worms which pierce through the intestines* without injuring them is stated in the Misc. Cur., Year 5, Obs. 45; also by BONETUS in his Book 3 of Sepulchretum, sive anatomia practica, Part 16, Obs. 12. That others again, piercing through the said parts, cause death is mentioned by the same author in Obs. 13.

A whole bundle or *clump of worms*, expelled after severe abdominal pain, is mentioned by HILDANUS [l.c.], in Part 1, Obs. 57; *a fragment of a worm, 7 yards long*, expelled by a woman: Part 2, Obs. 73.

That *worms* are expelled *from the navel* is taught by FORESTUS [l.c.] in his Book 7, Obs. 35 and the Observa-
(24) tions of the first Part. Further the Acta Hafn., Year

1673, Obs. 74, state that *pinworms* are *the cause of tenesmus*. For this, see also Part 3, the 26th aphorism of HIPPOCRATES.

Worms have sometimes been found *in an inguinal swelling*, according to the testimony of the famous Misc. Cur.; see Year 6 in Part 12, Obs. 144.

These *animalcules* are found *in the lung*, *the pleura*, *the pericardium*, and other parts of the chest, as reported by the Danish authors [Acta Hafn.] in their Part 3, Obs. 56, and by FORESTUS [l.c.] in his 21st Book, Obs. 26 in Part 3.

Indeed, even *the heart is not free from worms;* about this, see Obs. 13 in the Misc. Cur., Years 9 and 10.

That there are *worms in the veins* is described by JOH. RHODIUS [Observationes medicae], Obs. 6 [read: 61?]; he also detected them in the iliac arteries, see Obs. 61 [read: 62?].

PETRUS BORELLUS [l.c.] tells of animalcules having the form of a whale, which are present in the blood. See his Obs. 4 in Part 3.

FORETUS [read: FORESTUS] [l.c.] alleges that fever patients contain worms; see his Book 7, Obs. 36, Part 1.

KIRCHERUS [De peste] states them to be the causes or instruments of the plague.

RHODIUS [l.c.] mentions *an extremely big worm* and calls it the *cause of a protracted illness and death* in his Part 3, Obs. 64.

(25) It has been said above where HILDANUS [l.c.] and others found *worms*, *e.g.* *in the gall-bladder*, *the urinary bladder*, and elsewhere. But the Misc. Cur. report them in the *kidneys*, see Year 3, Obs. 405.

As nearly all authors who write about the symptoms of the diseases bring forward their observations on the urine, there are too many to mention them all who have found *worms* therein. Among all these it may suffice to mention the Misc. Cur., Years 3 and 4, Obs. 156; Year 3, Obs. 77; Year 6, Obs. 31. PECHLINUS [l.c.], Book 2, Obs. 18. The Acta Hafn., Part 5, Obs. 21. BONETUS in his aforementioned book, Obs. 33. TULP [l.c.], Book 2, Chapter 43. See also the Misc. Cur. under the word *Termites*.

Vermiform [according to the Latin edition] *blood* excreted with the urine is mentioned by BONETUS [l.c.] in his Obs. 34, Part 29 of Book 3; and also *an animalcule resembling a sow-bug, ejected alive with the urine*, in Obs. 35. Further *a worm ejected from the urinary bladder by a nursing woman* in Obs. 33.

The *worms* are also present *in the uterus;* about this, see Obs. 7 of Years 9 and 10, and Obs. 24 of Year 8, Part 2 [according to the Latin edition in Misc. Cur.]. In the *collum uteri* [according to the Latin edition] they are found by FORESTUS [l.c.], Book 21, Obs. 37 in the Scholium.

Worms in the legs, *the scrotum*, and *a tumour and bladder full of worms* are mentioned by the Misc. Cur., Years 3 and 4, Obs. 173, and also Year 7, Obs. 16.

In scabies and varioles they are described by BORELLUS [l.c.], Obs. 72.

In pustules, varioles, and the whole of the body: RHODIUS (26)
[l.c.], Obs. 64, Part 3.

A wholly wormy man (alas! that only this disease were somewhat rare!) is reported by the Danes in their [Acta Hafn.] Part 3, Obs. 11.

Severe symptoms caused by *mites* are reported by HILDANUS [l.c.], Obs. 96, as well as by BONETUS [l.c.] in his last Obs., Part 35: a *constant production of worms, from infancy to a great age.* Observations *about aged worms of different forms, big and small worms, and other animalcules* in all parts of the body are to be found. The dispute, or rather the argument, will now have to concern the question of whether these animalcules, which are admitted to be found in the parts of living human bodies, can or cannot be causes of diseases and their symptoms, the more so because, amongst others, TH. KERKRING, a man who has gained a great reputation in anatomy and medicine, doubts it, when on p. 177 in his [Specilegium anatomicum] Obs. 93 he tries to demonstrate the uncertainty of the opinion that is formed about things in anatomy by means and with the aid of magnifying glasses. He deduces this uncertainty: 1. from the smallness of the sharp centre of the field of

view; 2. from the change of colour; 3. from the alternate inspection of several parts, so that what now seems to
(27) be separate in reality is united, nay, united physically. But after having highly commended a certain magnifying glass and its maker, B. SPINOZA, he adds these words: *by means of this my admirable instrument I saw very wonderful things, viz. that the intestines, the liver, and all the tissue of the other intestines are filled with an infinite number of tiny animalcules; however, a person who considers that a house which is inhabited is clean and bright, but nevertheless wears away through the constant maintenance of those who inhabit it, will tend to doubt whether these animalcules spoil or maintain these parts through their continuous movement.*

Although I am not unaware what great acceptance, credence, and confidence the unfounded reputations of experience, example, and reports of so-called happenings and so on have received and kept not only among the common people, but unfortunately also among some prominent persons, I will not now oppose or cite any authors who deny or affirm that diseases and their symptoms are caused by worms and other animalcules in the human body. For, to express my opinion both frankly and respectfully, I think that any experience, observation, and example will never be applicable, unless at best somewhat in general, in particular.

Firstly, one never sees two cases – what do I say: Cases? one never sees two things – which are the same in every respect. On the basis of this statement I once said – and some people were pleased by it:

ALL THINGS ARE DIVINE, (28)
BECAUSE OF THEIR INFINITE VARIETY

Apply this to the medical art, then in my view the time of year, age, sex of the patient, mode of living, site of the defects, greater or lesser severity of the illness and the defect, and further many other circumstances will argue against the comparability and applicability of one observation to another case.

Secondly, few people and even fewer physicians and surgeons are found who are willing or have the courage to confess their errors, for the benefit of their fellowmen.

Thirdly: if it happened that after reasonable examination two cases very closely resembling each other were found, then I ask (in my view: with good reason): does one [have to] conclude reasonably from this an irrefutable truth and a resultant law that this always happens and this or that always has to be done first? I think not. Add to this:

Fourthly, no one should or may rely on witnesses in the medical and surgical arts. If this were done and everything for which witnesses could be found were true, all the miracles ever invented by the Papists for the adornment of their market would be true. If this

were done, on the evidence and assurances of a frightened or ignorant person one would have to assume a thousand follies to be true and charlatans would have
(29) to be preferred to wise physicians and sensible surgeons.

Fifthly: What credence is to be attached to reports of matters from which people derive profit or loss, according as they tell these matters? What will not many people, and certainly many physicians, do for profit? To say (and yet to lie withal): *I have cured this person of deafness with this instrument and that person of the falling sickness with that medicament*, is quite possible, until one seeks out these cured people and finds they are not cured at all or quite the reverse. Briefly, I keep to the rules of reason, using them as much as possible, employing my external senses and their aids, like a messenger for a letter, a tool for work, light for visibly distinguishing things which are already different, and so on. And I firmly believe that all diseases (I am not speaking of outwardly inflicted injury) are to be found first in the fluid parts, secondly in the ducts through which the latter flow, and thirdly in the parts into which they are conveyed; that further, more often than we think, animals are the cause of the poor condition of these three parts, their obstructed movement, and the results thereof, and I deny explicitly that the blood and the bile have ever been made or composed as many people describe. Commonly these parts and substances are incriminated, commonly they and their poor condition are called the causes of diseases. Of the first there is too much or too little; now too salt, now too sticky; (30) now too sour, now too watery; now too thick, now too thin. Of the second there is too much or too little; they are too tough or not tough enough; too bitter or not properly bitter; now combined and mixed too closely with the blood, now not closely enough; now burnt, now not boiled enough. All this talk will serve, and why not? The *visit* is rounded off by it, gets its *form*, and the quack doctor, *visiting* the patient, gets his money.

Anyone who wants to see the representation of such A „RAADSHEER" WITH A P IN THE MIDDLE OR IN FRONT, in a descriptive poem, should read the 7th Character of the Lord of ZUYLICHEM [CONSTANTIJN HUYGENS], but should not mingle among this crowd honest and learned men who, following the footsteps of reason and virtue, please God and men becasue of their wisdom and record of service performed in good faith for their suffering fellows. They know from the form, the constitution, the movement, that the blood cannot be salt or sour, the bile not burnt or watery; that the admixture of other substances does not change any part of its nature; they do not seek causes of diseases in fluids and organs which are not and never were present in the places where the disease is assumed to have originated; they are able and willing to understand that animalcules,

though they do not see them emerging in their thousands and several fathoms and feet long and thick, nor
(31) always, from the noses and ears of patients and dead bodies, may inflict diseases and injuries on the person in whom they are present; indeed, they will admit that, because animalcules can be found in all parts of the body, they also can and probably do cause illness in all parts of the body.

I have always found it takes more time to examine and become acquainted with the diseases and their causes than to cure or alleviate them after I had found them; indeed, I even look upon those things which are frequently alleged to be the causes of something as their consequences and effects. Thus, people call a watery tumour in the abdomen, an ulcer in the lung or the liver, a swelling in the groin, and so on, when found in dead bodies, the causes of the disease and of death, without reflecting that they are the consequences of previously broken, clogged, or otherwise injured ducts and impeded movements of certain fluids, and without investigating by what cause, in what place, when, and in what way these occurred or could occur. This is why for one and the same defect one person is seen to use medicaments full of volatile salt, another such as have an earthy and solid composition. But I will discuss this at greater length on another occasion, lest I digress too much from my subject-matter. In fact, I think I have

shown sufficiently how some animalcules get into human bodies. Now I imagine that the way in which they can injure, torment, and destroy them and thus be the causes of diseases and their symptoms, and even of (32)
death, is that these animalcules, which are sometimes found together in thousands,

firstly, extend excessively the parts which they inhabit, through the growth of their little bodies as well as the multiplication of their kind;

secondly, by breaking these parts by biting into and through them, these organs thus losing their function wholly or partly;

thirdly, by piercing into and through and insinuating themselves into ducts and places, the delicate texture of these ducts suffering from this;

fourthly, through fermentation of the saps, *viz.* when they impede and hinder their passage and discharge;

fifthly, by absorbing for their nourishment and growth the fluids, saps, and substances which are destined for the nourishment and growth or production and use of certain parts;

sixthly, by casting their excrements, eggs, young, and dead bodies between and into the parts, whose movement is thus impeded, which entails fatal consequences.

Several more ways of causing injury might be added, but I trust that these will suffice to give some idea of others as well.

Now the person who knows and uses a medicament which, without injuring the parts of the body, prevents
(33) these animalcules from gnawing, creeping about, and whatever else has been mentioned above, kills them or expels them while alive from the body, acts safely in this respect as to his prescription and cure. But even if it be admitted that the disorders of the fluid parts and thus of the blood and admixed substances, whether the disorder were conceived to consist in their condition or their motion, can cause certain diseases and their symptoms, will it therefore be called unreasonable to prove that also animalcules, mixed with them and indeed found in the solid parts, can cause certain diseases and their symptoms? Of the former, more words and of the latter, more solid proofs can be produced. It would therefore be more fair that those persons who always and solely rely upon their experiences should be guided by the latter, into which they ought to inquire first, to wit the reasons.

I should now speak further of the medicaments required above in general and in particular if it were not for the fact that I fear I have already transgressed the law of modesty, the title of this treatise, and the scope of an epistle devoted only to one purpose; indeed, that I am detaining you too long from your occupations, with matters which do not properly belong to your work, by prolonging the argument beyond the require-

ments of a letter and adding other things according to my experiences about these animalcules. But you as well (34)
as anyone who will ever take the trouble to read this letter will no doubt be able to take this in good part when recognizing that I have done this only for the advantage of the medical art and as an incentive to zealous investigators of the still concealed knowledge of many things, the number of which is truly unlimited. I will also, at the first opportunity, communicate to you courteously my ideas concerning the Fallopian tubes and other adjacent parts, on which you do me the honour to write.

Leyden, the 21st of March,
in the year 1698.

FACSIMILE

BRIEF

VAN

G: BIDLOO,

AAN

ANTONY van LEEUWENHOEK;

VVegens de dieren, welke men zomtyds in de lever der Schaapen en andere beesten vind.

Gedrukt Te DELFT, by HENRIK van KROONEVELT, Boekverkooper. 1698.

G. BIDLOO;

VVenscht den vermaarden Heere, ANTONI van LEEUVVENHOEK, vordering, genoegen en eere by zijnnen yver, in het onderzoeken der dierelijke Licchaamen en andere stoffen.

MYN HEER;

UWe heusche Brieven, Vrindelijk onthaal en aangenaame Vertoogen van veele weetenswaardige zaaken, verplichten my, de volgende waarneeming, over welke ons gesprek onlangs is geweest, UE. gedienstelijken aan te bieden en wel te meerder, om dat ik, ook door uwe eygene aanteekeningen en beschouwingen geheel en al van des zelfs waarheid, ben verzeekerd geworden.

Na dat ik, nu by toeval, dan by toeleg, veelmaalen in den lever der menschen en beesten, verscheidene ziektens, gezwellen, steenen, stoffen en wel bizonderlijken, in die van de schaapen, een geslacht van dieren hadden gevonden, wier benaaming, (Wurmen) beschrijving en afbeelding my niet, of immers gantsch weinig, met hun maakzel scheen over een te koomen, benaarstigde ik my, het zelve te onderzoeken: maar hebbende altijd de haatelijke gewoonte van den arbeid van andere kleen te achten, verfoeit, zach ik, alvoorens iets ter zaake te zeggen, naar, wat mannen van naam, geleerdheid en naarstigheid hier in en omtrent moggen ontdekt hebben: onder hen, om niet alom en als in het wilde heen te zoeken, doorblade ik de Schrijvers der laatere en onzer tijden en bevond, dat de nooit genoech geroemde FABRITIUS HILDANUS, in het 1ste. Deel zijnner Heelkundige aanmerkingen, op het 74ste. Blad, vraagd, *Wat 'er zeldzaamer? wat 'er verwonderlijker is? dan dat 'er Wurmen in den galblaas gevonden worden:* bevestigende nochtans het zelve, door het zeggen en gezach van den geloofwaardigen Heere GALENUS WIERUS, in zijnnen Brief, den 16den. Juny des Jaars 1602, uyt Dusseldorp geschreeven.

De Franszen (men zie hunne dagaanteekeningen, onder het opschrift van *Journal des Sçavans*, op het

Jaar

Jaar 1668. uytgegeeven) bezich in het nader onderzoek van den buys, waar door de gal in den pijp des galblaas gevoerd werd, vonden in de galpijpen van een ſchaap deeze zoo genaamde Wurmen en wilde eenige uyt hen, zijnde ter dier tijd eene algemeene vreeze te Parijs voor de Peſtziekte, mogelijk het geſchrift van ATH. KIRCHERUS over de Peſtziekte in het Jaar 1658. uytgegeeven, geleezen hebbende, in bedenken geeven; of deeze dierkens niet wel voorbooden van die droeve quaale mogten zijn, wijl CORN. GEMMA, van iets diergelijks, omtrent het Jaar 1562. in Holland voorgevallen, ſpreekt; willende, dat de meenigvuldige ziektens en zwaare ſterftens der beeſten, voorteekenen van die der menſchen zijn. Zy vergelijken de gedaante van het diertje, by die van het Glidkruyt, het welk in de weijen groeit, beſchrijven het zelve wyders aldus: *Zy zijn plat, eywijs en een weinig puntig naar het eene uyteÿnde, van omtrek, hebbende het hoofd aan het andere gedeelte een weinig uytſteekende, het welk het ſteeltje van het blad verbeeld. Zy zijn blankachtig op den buijk, op den rug met veel vlekjens en draadtjens van een donkere bruijnne verf bezet, het welk hun naar den Tong doed gelijken. Het Hoofd heeft een Snuyt, welke van een kleen gat, behalven een ander, het welk veel grooter en omtrent het midden, naar beneden gevonden werd, doorboord is.* Zy doen daar de volgende afbeelding en deezen uytleg by;

1. Verbeeld het dier, op den rug; 2. op den buyk, leggende, 3. het blad van het bovengenoemde kruijd, gelijk het BAUHINUS beſchrijft.

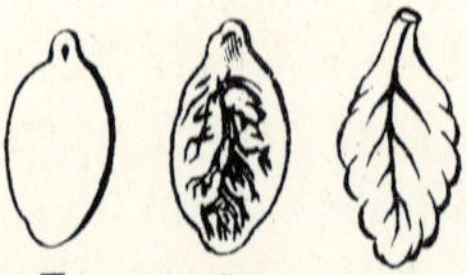

1. 2. 3.

Vorder voegen zy 'er niets toe; dan een algemeen vertoog van de onzeekerheid der voorbeduydingen, voorzeggingen en voorteekenen van de Peſtziekte.

Wat de Heeren BARTHOLINUS, FABRITIUS, HAUPTMANNUS, TARDINUS en andere van deeze en zommige andere gediertens zeggen, vind men te zaamen gebragt, in de naauwkeurige dagregiſters van het Hoogduytſche konſtgenoodſchap, op het Jaar 1670. het 128ſte. en 1675, 1676. in de aanteekeningen van den Heer FROMANNUS, op het 249ſte. en verdere bladen. Omtrent de zelve tijd, te weeten, in het Jaar 1671. heeft ook de Heer FRANCISCUS REDI, alom door zijne verdienſten bekend, in zijn verhandeling van de bloedeloozе dieren, op het 302de. blad, van deeze diertjens

jens geſprooken en aldus hunne gedaante uytge-beeld.

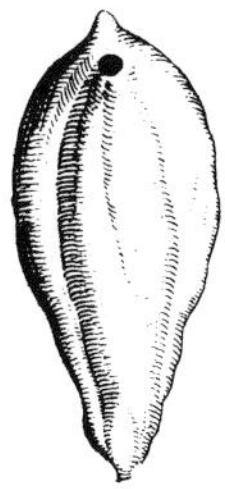

Vergelijkende de zelve by het zaad van Cauwoerde, of het kleen myrtheblad met een ſteeltje; zeggende wyders, *dat zy melkachtig wit en met uyt den geele groene pijpen voorzien zijn; een mond, of gat, niet wijd van den ſtaart, in de vlakte van den buyk, hebben: dikmaals niet alleen in den galblaas; maar ook in alle de vaten van den lever, de ſlagaderen uytgezonderd, der ſchaapen gevonden werden.* Wat van dit alles, naar mijnne bevinding, aan te neemen zy, gelieve UE. in het vervolg te zien.

Eyndelijken vond ik, dat ook de Heer FRED. RUYSCH op het 84ste. blad zijnner aanmerkingen, van de voorgemelde diertjens gewag maakt: maar hoe verre zijnne uytbeelding van de waarheid en de gedaante deezes diers (want behalven deeze en waar het zelve van hem in den lever der ſchaapen gevonden is, zegt hy 'er weinig van) wijkt, zal blijken, wanneer men deeze zijnne uytbeelding, tegen de

'E

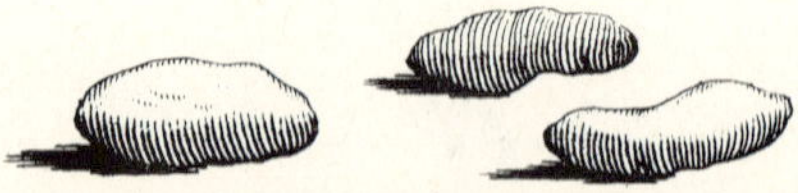

waare en de mijnne zal gelieven te vergelijken; zullende, zoo ik vertrouw, geen mensch, deeze afbeelding voor die van een dier, als niets hebbende, het welk naar een leevend schepzel zweemt; maar veel eerder voor die van een klierweezen, of andere stoffe, moeten aanzien. Hy zegt nochtans, by aanwijzing van den Letter E. *Wurmen uyt den huys der galblaas en galpijpen van een schaap genoomen.*

Om, in begrijpelijke schikking, van het genoemde diertje te handelen, zal ik mijnne aanmerkingen en waarneemingen, eerstelijken, omtrent des zelfs licchaam aanvangen; ten 2^{den}. de plaatzen daar het gevonden werd; ten 3^{den}. der zelver getal, wording, voortteeling en ten vierden aanwijzen, dat deeze en andere diertjes, in den lever en andere deelen des licchaams zich onthoudende, de oorzaaken van zommige ziektens en hunne gevolgen kunnen zijn.

I. Belangende de gedaante, omtrek en gelijkenis van deeze diertjes, nu (boven de voorgemelde gelijkenissen) by het blad van het penningkruyd, dan

by

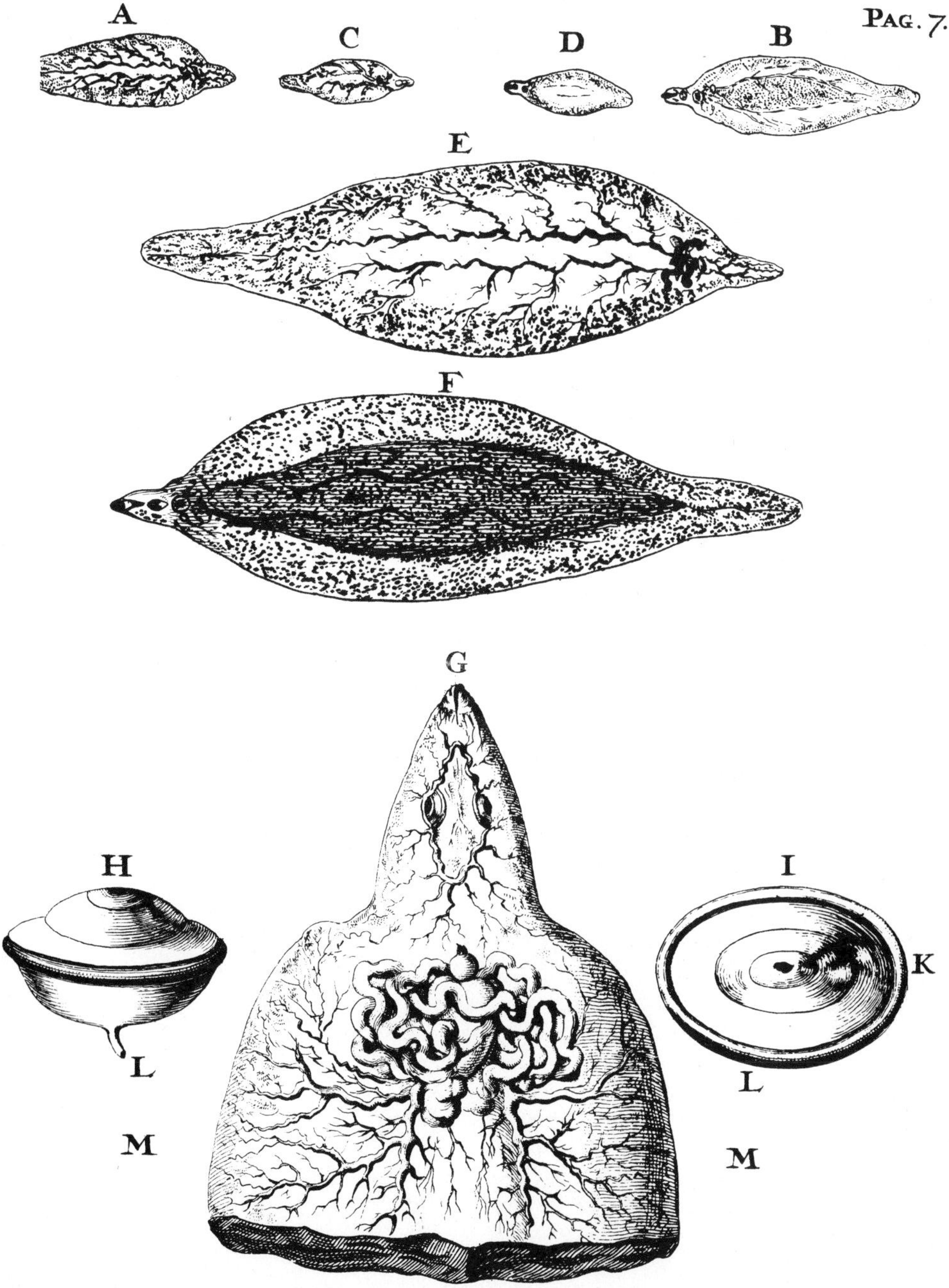
A
C
D
B
E
F
G
H
I
K
L
L
M
M

by een Bloedzuyger vergeleeken, de zelve is onzen visch Tong, of Both, in het kleene, zeer naar koomende; als te zien is, in de eerste afteekening; verbeeldende A. een deezer diertjes, naar de groote, welke men gemeenelijk van hen bevind, op de bultige, ofte zyde des rugs; B. het zelve omgekeerd en alzoo van den buyk aan te zien, C. vertoond een jong van de zelve, op de eerste, D. op de twede wijze aan te schouwen. Onder de aanwijzing van de Letteren E. en F. vind men het diertje, by vergrooting van het geheele licchaam, op de eene en andere zijde afgeteekend.

Men ziet ze zelden leevende, naardien deeze ziekte uyterlijken niet te kennen en het beest, dat de zelve onderwurpen is, zomtijds vet en gezond voortkomt, werd alzoo de lever niet, dat dan naâr den dood, onderzocht; kunnende ook deeze diertjes geen koude, of bywerp van ander vocht lijden. Ik heb ze nâa veel maalen by het daar toe bizonderlijken aangestelde slagten gebleeven te hebben, leevende en laatst den 13den. Maart in groote meenigte, gelijk ten zelven tijde een geslacht van korte, dikke Wurmen in den lever van een Kat, gezien. Wanneer zy beginnen koud te werden en aldus hunne beweeging verliezen, hervatten zy de zelve, als zy in een warme hand gehouden, of wel den lever in warm water gelegt werd. Hunne beweeging is, gelijk die van de bovengemelde Visschen, dat is, golvende, werdende de kanten van het lichaam voortgaande omgeworpen en alzoo het hoofd eerst ingehaald, het licchaam verbreed en daar nâa, in de lengte, uytgerekt

rekt. Hun verf is bruyngeel, de buyk gantſch plat en veel bleeker dan de rug: voorts is hun huyd ruw, met ſtippen bezet en zoo doorzichtig, dat men er de ingewanden en vaten ter weederzijden door heen kan onderkennen. Het hoofd hebben ze (zie de afteekening by vergrooting onder den Letter G.) uyt den ſpitze platrond, den mond uytpuylende in de hoogte, open zijnde, eyrond, by naar op de wijze van een Karper. De oogen (zie als boven de Letters H. en I.) welke zeer uytſteeken, werden met een K. kraakbeenachtigen ring omtoogen en zijn, gelijk in veele platte Viſſchen, niet ter weder; maar op eene zijde van des hoofd verdeeling geplaatſt.

Het hert is zoo kort aan het hoofd en wederom de darmen zoo naauw aan het zelve gelegen, dat ik twijfel of'er wel iets is, waar door het hoofd van het vervolg des lichaams, het welk nochtans den meeſten dieren eygen is, onderſcheiden werd. Van het hert ſpreijen zich twee vaten, door het geheele lichaam uyt; laatende een wijde tuſſchenplaats in het midden van den rug, naar des zelfs lengte, op de wijze als te zien is, onder de Letter L., tuſſchen hen loopen M. gantſch dunne pijpjens, of draadjens, waar in men geen vocht kan onderkennen. Ik vinde in de eerſte twee zoorten van vocht, dat is, in zommige bruyngeel; ja zomtijds purpurachtig, in andere bleekgroen, beide altijd ſlijmachtig zijnde, vloeijende nochtans (ook wanneer het dierken dood is en by het achterſte gedeelte werd opgeheven) naar het hert en wederom van daar, wanneer men

het

het hoofd optild , naar het achtereynde des lichaams. Eenige Heeren verwonderden zich , dat dit heen-en wedervloeijen , als de diertjens leeven, veel traager toegaat (daar nochtans het vocht dunner in hen , by hun leven, dan nâa hun dood is) dan wel wanneer zy dood zijn : maar gedenkende aan de afdragende buyzen en de voortperſzende beweeging van het hert, wierd hen de reeden en daar nâa, de uytwerking dês vertoogs klaar en duydelijk.

De darmen hebben hunnen uytgang , of navel, dus noemd men, door een quaade gewoonte, die opening in de viſſchen, op de rechter zyde des licchaams, zeer kort onder het hoofd: weshalven de zelve zeer kort in een gedrongen leggen. Een klompken uyt den zwarten , aan het begin der darmen geplaatſt, neeme ik voor den lever.

Tuſſchen dit en de darmen, vinde ik, in alle de dieren, welke ik onderzocht heb, den ontelbaaren hoop der eyronde deeltjens, waar van U. E. in zynnen Brief ſpreekt en ervaare als hy, dat honderden van hen te zaamen gevoegd , naauwelyks de groote van een grof zand uytmaakende, een flaauw rood vertoonen. Zy komen my voor den kuyt , of de eyeren deezer dieren voor ; maar wat naarſtigheid ik ook aangewend heb , my is noch niet gelukt, geheel zeeker elks diers kunne te onderſcheyden: zynde mêermaalen in twyfel , komt my, voor het naaſte aan de waarheid, voor, dat zy van dat geſlacht der dieren zyn, in welke men eene dubbele kunne ziet ; of dat my, tot nu toe, geen manneken in de hand gevallen is. Hoe verre nu het getal der wyfjens, dat van de mannekens in zommige waterdieren overtreft, bevind men onder andere in de Schelvisſchen. Of nu deeze dieren, water-wurmen, of visſchen moeten genoemd werden, diend ter zaake niet, wyl men dit ook in dieren, die op het Land leeven, als zyn ſlakken en andere, ervaard. De kleenheid des licchaams doed'er ook af, noch toe: want daar zyn veel geſlachten van water- en land dieren, hen in groote en aanwas al om gelyk: Ja duyzende, duyzendmaal kleen'er en van verſcheydene gedaante, ziet men'er daagelyks, zelfs in het regenwater. Ik verzoek dat U. E. op het voorgemelde, zyn aanmerking mag believen te laaten gaan. Ik bevinde ook, gelyk U. E. my geliefde mede te deelen, dat zich overal, waar men jonge van deeze dieren ziet, veele der bovengenoemde eyronde deeltjens, in het vocht, zynde diepgeverfde gal, waar in zy leggen, opdoen, welke, hoe kleen zy ook zyn, nochthans alle van eene en zelve gedaante en doorſchynnende bevonden werden.

De ſtaart, of het uyteynde, ſchoon met het geheele licchaam overeenkomende, is echter veel tederder, dan eene van al de andere uyterlyke deelen, breekende op de minſte ruwe aanraaking.

De plaatzen, waar ik het zelve, tot noch toe, gevonden heb, zyn alleen de vaten, buyzen en vergaaderplaatzen, ten dienſte van de gal geſchikt; meeſt zynze echter in de galbuyzen, welke, in dit geval, alomme; toch boven maaten en met zwaare bulten, kringen, bochten en huyskens, wier holtens middelyn

delyn diklmaal 1. en ½ duymbreet uytgezet is, uyt-steeken, ter plaatze, daar men deeze dieren op een gepakt vind leggen; zynde ook die plaatzen kraakbeenachtig hart. In de kleene galpypen leggen zy naar de lengte en zomtyds wel dryvoudig in een gerold en meene ik, dat hier door veele, omtrent der zelver gedaante, bedrogen zynde, hen, als langwerpigronde wurmen, hebben beschreeven: toch hoe zeer in een gewonden, spreijen zy zich nochthans, ook naa de dood, in warm water gewurpen, straks naar hunne vlakte uyt; maar veranderen ook voort eenigzins (te weeten bleek werdende) van verwe.

Zelden ziet men deeze dieren, zonder dat'er te gelyk ook, in den lever, gezwellen, of zweeren gezien werden: maar hoe veele, hoe weinige, hoe kleen, of groot ook de dieren waaren, ik hebbe nooit de bloedvaten, geene uytgezonderd, van hunne gewoone gedaante, noch het bloed in de zelve veranderd, veel minder de dieren in hunne holtens gevonden: houdende de zenuwen hunne algemeene loop, gestrektheid en zaamenstel in volkomenheid; vinde ik de watervaten, door het geheele licchaam van hunne gewoone staat verschillende, zynde zommige boven maaten uytgespannen, andere geheel plat; ja naauwlyks zichtbaar en in dat geval, is de holligheid van den buyk vol water; het klierweezen van den lever, in zynne tusschenwytens, zeer van een en uytgezet, ieder klier met vocht gevuld en doordrongen, onderscheidelyken zichtbaar en van zyn gebuurklier, als afgezonderd; zelf het buytenvlies van de lever, dikker en harder, dan naar gewoonte. Het zal zeer aanneemelyk zyn, dat deeze dieren nooit in het weezen des levers, of des zelfs bloed-vaten huysvesten, wanneer men bereedenkaveld, dat de zelve, of van buyten, dat niemand beweeren zal willen, of wel door de bloed- gal, of waterpypen, daar in moesten gebragt werden.

Eerstelyken, de slagaderen zwaar van zaamenstel, voorts zeer eng; ia wel zoo eng, omtrent hunne uyteynden, in den lever zynde, dat de zelve geene deezer dierkens kunnen omvangen (ik zwyge alhier de tegenreeden, uyt de beweeging van het bloed en andere oorzaaken af te leyen) besluite ik, met den Heere Redi, onmoogelyk te zyn, dat de zelve in de slagaderen hun verblyf en aanwas kunnen bekomen: maar achte nochthans (behoudens zyn Ed: groote naam) tegen zyn Ed: gevoelen, dat de zelve ook in de andere bloedvaten niet zyn: want werden zy (dit beweerd zyn Ed:) in de galblaas geteeld, booren zy, van daar doorgekroopen, al bytende, door den gemeenen galbuys en wederom van daar, door en in de bloedbuyzen, zoo moest men alom uytgestort, of uytstortend bloed zien, het welk ik noch nooit hebbe ervaaren. Dat zy aldaar, in getal vermeerderd, al wederom door de bloedvaten knaagen, dus in het klierweezen des levers dringen en aldaar hollekens maaken, is, behalven de onwaarschynlykheid, ook tegen de bevinding; werdende de alderkleenste galpypen, wanneer'er deeze dieren in zyn, ook zelfs omtrent den dunsten ommetrek des levers, zoodaanig uitgezet, vergroot en verwyderd, dat des zelfs klierweezen met het buytenvlies vereenigd werd,

zynde

zynde in de hollekens geene de minste stoffe, welke naar bloed gelykt, te vinden.

Het getal deezer dieren is, gemeenelyken, groot; toch onzeeker en naar de dieren meerder, of minder tyd, tot hun voorteeling gehad hebben; hebbende ik uyt eene lever 870. geheele, behalven veele gebrookene en in het doorsnyden en uyttrekken geschondene; uyt eene andere, maar 10, of 12, kunnen haalen. Men vindze in veel'erhande geslachten van beesten. Jagers, op de veluwe, zeggen my, de zelve in Herten, Wilde varkens en ander grof en kleen wild, gevonden te hebben. In Kalven heb ik ze dikmaals en in een jongen Stier, een pink, voor weinig dagen, toch uyt den groenen zwart van verf, gezien. Dat zy in de Schaapen van den baarmoeder af, in lammeren, eens en meermaalen verjaarde; ja verouderde schaapen gevonden werden, is veelen en U Ed: al lang, bekend geweest. Ik hebbe meenigmaalen op en omtrent den lever der Menschen wurmen; maar van eene geheele andere gedaante en maakzel gevonden: hoewel ik, als nu nader kennisse van de bewuste diertjens hebbende en bizonderlyken, hoe zy zich in eèn kunnen rollen, my durf verbeelden, de zelve eenige jaaren geleeden, in den lever van een Mensch, gezien te hebben: toch zal, alvoorens dit te bevestigen, alomme gelegenheid zoeken, om hier van (ik verzoek het U Ed: ook) de waarheid te ontdekken. Noopende deezer dieren, wording, eerstvoortbrengende oorzaak, stoffe en voortteeling, welke zommige Schrijvers uyt verrotting, bederving, gebrek van zout, ongemaatigdheid

tigdheid van vocht, warmte en andere zinlooze gedachten, woorden en hoedanigheden, gelyk, dat zy eens uyt verrotte ſtof voortgebragt zynde, *Multiplicativi ſui mediante, ſive operante facultate foventrice*, zyn en andere beuzelachtige grillen meer, poogen af te leyen: ik verwerp deeze alle, ſtelle vaſt dat deeze dieren, gelykerwys al wat *dierlyken*, of beroerlyken leeft, uyt zyns gelyke en dus uyt eyeren, zaad, kuyt, kortom, ſtof hem in zynne eerſte wording gelykvormig en even eens van geſtel, voortkomt; achtende, dat de eeuw, waar in wy leeven, te verre in de kenniſſe der taſt-en zichtbaare (ik zwyge andere) zaaken; te verre op den goeden grond van reedenkaavelen; te verre op den weg van wel onderzoeken gevorderd is, dan dat men zich en andere, met dien vermuften en verzuften ouderwyven en quylender kinderen klap, beeter, op den voet van het onverlichte heidendom, onder een ſprookje van een verzierden Droomgod, of eenen Lallus aan den wieg, dan onder een hebbelyk geſprek van ook maar middelbaar verſtandige menſchen voegende, langer zou durven, of kunnen op-en gaande houwen. Ik zoude op het boven gemelde voorwerp langer ſtaan, was deeze ſtofte, voor weinig tyd, in het breede, door Mr. C. van STEENEVELD, onder de redenering wegens DE WURM-ZWEEREN niet verhandeld geworden: in welken hy, wederleggende de 64^{ſte}: der aanmerkingen door den Hr: FR: RUYSCH beſchreeven, den zelven zonneklaar van de voorgemelde waarheid overtuygt. U E: zie het voornoemde geſchrift, van het 9de, tot het 18de, blad en hy zal'er zynnen naam geèerd, zynne

zynne bevindingen, ter grooter aandrang van bewijs, ingevoegd vinden,

De gelegenheid, by welken U. E. meent, gelyk hy al in het Jaar 1679. aan het Koninklyk Konſtgenoodſchap in Engeland ſchreef, dat deeze dierkens en hunne eyeren in de ſchaapen komen (van andere diertjens en hunne eyeren, zal men het zelve moeten onderſtellen) naamelyken, dat de zelve in vochtige Zoomer-en Herſſt tyden, uit het aardryk opwellende, met het vocht, waar in zy leeven, of komen, ingedronken werden, vinde ik, (hebbende my des wegen, door Boeren, beeſte-weyers en Slagters doen berichten) zeer waarſchijnlyk, dan (het zy met U. E. believen gezegd) geenzints, dat de zelve door maag en darmen boorende, uyt de holligheid van den buyk, in de vaten van den lever zouden dringen, aldaar voortteelen en in de maag en darmen openingen maakende, de werkende oorzaaken zijn, dat (uyt die gàtjens) den grooten magt des waters, welke zomtijs in de holligheid van den Buijk gevonden werd, werd uytgeſtort en uytzijpeld: want komen zy, nu al dieren zynde, in de maag en darmen, kunnen zy al door de zelve booren, zoo zullen zy ook door de vliezen van de andere ingewanden, aan en by de voornoemde gelegen, als het klierbedde, nieren, milt, zekerlijken kunnen booren en (dat ik noch nooit gezien heb) in de zelve gevonden werden.

U E: doe hier ten 2den by, dat zy dan allomme zichtbaar genoech zouden zyn en ook immers, ten minſten in den maag, of darmen moeten (dat ook niet geſchied) gevonden werden

Ten

Ten 3den, al boorden zy door de voorgenoemde deelen, zoo zou'er, gijl, of vocht, in dunheid gijl gelyk, moeten uytvloeijen. Anderzints zou men, was het vocht grover, de gàten in die ingewanden moeten ontdekken. Ik heb, om hier van de waarheid te onderzoeken, de maag en darmen van een Schaap, met deeze quaale, ten uyterften, gequeld, toen zy warm waaren gedrukt, doorzocht, naamaals de zelve in warm water gehouwen, met warm water gevuld, wederom in het laagfte gedeelte warme brandewijn en eyndelijken quiqzilver gegooten, als toen, bewoogen, gedout en herdoud, bezien, behandeld op alle (my bedenkelijke) wijzen; dan hebbe geene de minfte openingen in de zelve kunnen befpeuren. Dat de zelve uyt de 12 vingerigen darm, door de gemeene galweg, in de galblaas en galpijpen zouden kruijpen, daar hunne jongen teelen, &c: ftrijd te veel met het bekende geftel en werking, of gebruik deezer deelen; dan dat ik dit behoef te wederleggen.

De gedachten, welke U E: my, den 19den: January laaftleeden fchreef, omtrent het drinken van graftwater en fpijs bereiding voor de menfchen, dat, naamelijken, daar door veel dieren (ik verftâa waterdieren en hunne eijeren) in het licchaam van den menfch kunnen komen, gaan by my door; dan ftelle vaft, dat het water, het welk men in de holligheid van den buijk, als boven, in menfchen en beeften vind, alleenlijken uyt geborftene, gebrookene, of anderzints gefchondene watervaten, zijpeld; maar niet uyt de gatjens lekt, welke deeze dieren in den maag, of darmen maaken: maar begrijp ook met eene, dat zy dieren, de watervaten en der zelver begintzelen in den lever, schoon in de watervaten zelfs niet zijnde, kunnen breeken en schenden: zijnde, voor my, eene zeekere waarheid, dat het zaad, of de eyerkens van deeze en andere dieren (UE. zie hier op het 12de: en 13de: blad, in het geschrift van Mr. STEENEVELD) met het gijl, onder het bloed, met het bloed in den lever (ten opzichte van deeze diertiens in het bizonder) voorts in deezen alleen in de wegen en werktuygen van den gal kunnen komen, blijven, voortteelen en alzoo de gebuurdeelen scheuren en verbreeken.

Zy huysvesten eerstelijken niet, in de bloedvaten in het algemeen, noch ook in die van den lever, in het bizonder, als niets hebbende (ik zonder eeniger maate den poortader uyt) waar in en door zy van de algemeene bloedvaten, weezentlijken, verschillen. Ik zegge niet in de bloedvaten; zoo, om der zelver, als, des bloeds en der bygemengder sappen geduurige, eygene en voortgaande beweeging.

Ten 2^{den}, niet in de watervaten, om de voorgemelde reeden; der zelver engte en geduurige afvoering van vocht, uyt eene naauwe naar eene wijder plaatze.

Ten 3^{den}, niet in de zenuwen, als zynde geene pijpholle deelen, wier eynden in de holte der galbuyzen uyt- en open gaan.

Ten 4^{den}, niet in en tusschen het scheedevlies, den poortader en galpijpen omkleedende; sluytende het zelve alom zonder tusschenwijte en ook zelf geen opene pijpen hebbende , welke tot de galbuyzen, waar in zy dieren alleen gevonden werden , doorgaan.

Ten 5den , ook niet tusschen en in de plaatzen, alwaar slagader en ader , na eene onbepaalde takmaaking en verdeeling van der zelver stronk en voorts uyt grootere in mindere spranken, in de gedaante van een vlekje, by een komende , de klieren maaken ; zijnde ook deeze plaatzen zoo kleen en tot den overdragd van het bloed, als ook de scheiding des waters, aldus by uytnementheid genoemd en ten dienste des voedzels, voorts tot geduurige beweeging geschikt , is het niet te begrijpen, dat zy tot voortteeling van deeze dierkens zouden kunnen dienen.

Ten 6den, veel minder in het vlies, het welk den lever omkleed , ofte den strengader, nu al in een band veranderd, ofte ook in het pees- en vliesgestel, het welk den lever aan het middelrift bind: ik meene derhalven naar de reeden en uyt mynne ervaaring te mogen besluiten , dat deeze dieren alleen in de werktuijgen , buijzen en vergaaderplaatzen van den gal geteeld , vergroot en wederom in hun geslacht vermeerderd kunnen werden. Tot noch verder bewijs van dit gestelde , diene; eerstelijken, de overweeging, dat het zaad, de kuyt, of eyeren van deeze dieren , met het olijachtige gedeelte des gijls in het hier mede bezette beest, van het bloed in de werktuygen van den gal gebragt, aldaar kunnen aangezet werden en rusten, zynde de wanden dier vaten altijd met een slijmachtig en traag bewoogen werdende vochtigheid beslagen: men doe hier by, dat

dat de gal niet , gelijk het bloed, altijd in voortgaande beweeging is ; werdende des zelfs uytwerpend vat, na tusſchen des darms vliezen een weinig heen gevoerd te zyn, met een kring van ſpiervezelen geſloten; om naar vereyſch, nu toe, dan open te kunnen zyn.

Ten 2den: waar men deeze dieren, of hunne eyeren vind, zyn de galvaten in bulten uytgezet, hard en van verwe veranderd , hangende de dieren zelf zoo vaſt aan den vernoemden dikken gal, dat'er hunne licchaamtjens, nu al afgenoomen, nochtans alomme mede bezet zyn.

Ten 3den: het vocht, dat men hen ten monde en navel uytdrukt, is het zelve, dan alleen wat dunner, daar zy in leeven en van welks zommige deelen zy gevoed werden: maar wat wonder? ieder dier heeft zyn leefplaats en voedſtof in het bizonder, naar vereyſch van zyn geſtel. Zeeviſch ſterft in zoet, rievierviſch in zout water, een wurm in de lucht een vogel in de aarde en zoo voorts. Wat wonder (zegge ik dan) is het, dat dit dier, nu in het licchaam van een ander dier gevoerd , alleen in zyn leefplaats en leefſtof , of die'er meeſt mede overeenkomt, te weeten in de werktuijggen van den gal en in den gal zelfs, leeft , groeit, teeld en gevonden werd? derhalven achte ik het eene gantſch ongegronde leering, dat men, om wurmen en andere gediertens uyt de licchaamen der menſchen te drijven, hen alleen bittere geneeſmiddelen moet geeven: want ook immers ziet men het tegendeel in zommige wurmziektens: ten voorbeelde zy tandpijn; om welken te geneezen men honing, zuijker, of andere zoete ſtoffe aan de bedurvene tanden brengende, daar door en mede wurmen uyt de zelve haald en aldus de ziekte geneeſt.

Om nu aan te wijzen, dat deeze en andere dieren in den lever en andere plaatzen en deelen der lichaamen zich onthoudende, de oorzaaken van zommige ziektens en hunne bygaande toevallen zyn; weete men in het algemeen, dat'er naauwelijken ſtoffen te noemen zyn, in welke zomtijds geen dieren gevonden werden. Die hier van een kort begrip begeerd, leeze de aanteekening, door den Hr. PHILIPPÛS SCHAS VAN LEEUWENHEIMB, gedaan en door het Hoogduijtſche konſt genoodſchap, in hunne verzaameling der aanmerkenswaardige gevallen, onder die van het Jaar 1670, op het 34ſte: en volgende bladen gebragt: maar om kort te zyn, weete men, in het bizonder, ik zwyge van andere ſchepzelen, dat'er in den menſch geene zoo vloedige, of zoo vaſte deelen te noemen zyn (want eyndelijken behooren onze aanmerkingen in en omtrent andere dieren en ſtoffen, ten nutte van den menſch, te ſtrekken) in en omtrent welke, de aldoorſnuffelende naarſtigheid, zederd weinige Jaaren (men prijze U E. voorbeeld) geene leevende dieren ondekt heeft.

Ik wil (als ſtrijdende tegen de waarheid) niet beweeren, dat men altyd toonen kan, dat in alle ziektens, jeukten, hair-endouwurm, zweeren en gezwellen, dieren en noch wel die, oorzaaken van de zelve zyn: naardien ik weet, dat men uyt zommige puyſten een ſtoffe dringd, welke niets meerder gelijkt;

gelykt; toch niet minder, dan een wurmtie is. Zie hier een aanteekening van gevallen en plaatzen der menschelijke licchaamen, waar in dieren, wurmen en andere gedrogjens, door mannen van oordeel en naarstigheid gevonden zyn; want wilde ik een zaamenraapzel van de beuzelpraat, welke men op dit voorwerp zou kunnen vinden, omtrent deezer en anderer dieren wonderlijke vormwiszeling, voortteeking, kragt van byten en booren te voorschijn brengen, ik zou den tijd, U E. kennisse van deeze zaaken en myn geduld te kort doen.

Wurmen zyn dan *in het hoofd gevonden*; zie de voornoemde Hoogduytsche dagregisters. 1ste: 100. 2de: Jaar. aanmerck. 147. en het Jaar 3. aanmerk: 414. 2de: 100. op het Jaar 9. en 10. aanmerk: 50

Van veertig Maaywurmen, van een oude Vrouw, *door de neusgaten geloost*, na een zwaare hoofdscheelpijn geleeden te hebben, spreekt P. BORELLUS, in zyn geschrift der zeldzaame waarneemingen, zoo in de naareeden, als de 19. en 39ste: aanmerking.

Op het herde herszenvlies vondmen *een wurm*, zoo FORESTUS verhaald; in zyn 9de: Brief, de 4de: aanmerking van het eerste deel.

Van diergelyke meld HILDANUS; in de eerste 100, de 16de; zynner aanmerkingen; als ook van eene *door den neus geloost*, als boven, de 8ste: aanmerk.

Wurmen der oogen doed ons PECHLINUS, in zyn 2de: B. de 35ste: waarneeming, kennen.

Hoe de zelve *door den neus uytgeworpen* wierden,

 leest

leest men by FORESTUS, het 21. B. waarn: 26. van de 3de: verdeeling. De hoogduytsche dagRegisters 2de: 100. het 3de: Jaar. aanm: 99. by TULP het 4. B. het 12de: hooftstuk. P: BORELLUS, het 3de: 100. aanmerk: 45.

Hoe veel maal *wurmen in de ooren* gevonden werden, is te vinden, by de meergemelde hoogduytsche aanteekeningen, op het 3. en 4de: Jaar, waarn: 5. By FORESTUS, het 21ste: B. de 26. waarn: in het 12. B. waarn: 9. PLINUS, het 20. B. 14de: hoofdstuk: J. B. MONTANUS. waarn: 40.

Van *Tandpynwurmen*, spreekt PECHLINUS B. 2. waarn: 36.

Van *wurmen der tanden zelfs*, vind men een reeks gevallen aangeteekend, by de meermaal gemelde Hoogd: zie het Jaar 5. waarn: 192. het Jaar 9. en 10. waarn: 24 en 187. in de Deensche aanteek: het 5de: deel, de 108ste waarn: LEEUWENHOEK. dat'er *wurmen in het speegzel* zwemmen, beschrijven, neffens de duytsche, op het 9: en 10de: Jaar in de 130ste: aanteek: veele andere, zeggende HILDANUS in zyn eerstê deel, de 59 aanmerk: dat een meenigte der zelve *in het tandvleesch* huysvestende, de oorzaak des doods zyn geweest.

Uyt de ruggraat komen wurmen, volgens het verhaal der duytschers, zie op het 2de: Jaar, de 10de: aanteek: PETRUS BORELLUS vindze *op den Rug* en noemt hen, naar de plaats, *rugwurmen*, het 1ste: deel, de 89ste: waarn: niet alleen wurmen; maar *slakken* werden zomtyds door braaken uyt het licchaam gewurpen: zie als boven, de duytsche 85ste: waarn: in het

het eerſte deel, van het 3de: Jaar. Onbepaald is het getal der aanmerkingen, welke men vind van *wurmen ter maage uytgeſpoogen* : als by voorbeeld; de Hoogd: ſpreeken van de zelve op het 3de: Jaar de 258ſte: op het zelve en het 4de: Jaar waarn: 38. en 80. in het 2de: deel, het 4de: Jaar, waarn: 39. het 6de: Jaar, waarn: 33.

Van deeze, maar wit en langer, handeld FORESTUS, in het 21. B. de 26ſte: waarn. als ook ter zelver plaats, dat een oud man 'er 500. en een ander 300. hadde uytgeſpouwd.

Dat *Maagwalging door wurmen* werd veroorzaakt, beweeren de geneesheeren van Koppenhagen, in het 5de: deel hunner aanteekeningen, met de 34ſte: aanm:

Dat'er *wurmen* zyn, *die de darmen*, zonder ſchaade, *doorbooren*, ſtellen de hoogdt. vaſt, op hun 5de: Jaar. de 45ſte: aanm: ook BONETUS in zyn 3de: boek van de geneesk: der Noordſch: vol: de 16. verdeeling en aldaar de 12de: aanm: dat wederom andere, de zelve deelen doorboorende, den dood veroorzaaken, meld de zelve ſchrijver, in de 13de: waarn:

Van een geheel boſch, of *klomp van wurmen*, naa groote darmpyn, gelooſt, maakt HILDANUS gewag: in het 1ſte: deel, de 57ſte: aanmerk: van *een ſtuk van een wurm*, door een vrouw gelooſt, 7. *ellen lang* 2de: deel, de 73ſte: aanm:

Dat'er *wurmen uyt den navel* gedreeven werden, leerd ons FORESTUS, in zyn 7 B. waarn: 35. en de aanteek: der 1ſte: verdeeling: wyders de Deenſche aan-

tekeenaars

teekenaars op het Jaar 1673. aanm: 74 dat de *Maaywurmen oorzaak van den druploop* zyn. Zie hier ook op in het 3de: deel de 26ste: korte ſpreuk van HIPPOCRATES.

Wurmen vondmen ooit *in een lieſch buyl*, naar de getuygenis van de beroemde hoogdt: zie op het 6de: Jaar, in de 12de: verdeeling, de 144ste: aanmerking.

Deeze *dieren* vind men *in den long*, *het ribbevlies*, *hartezakje* en andere deelen van den borſt, gelyk dit, de deenſche ſchrijvers in hun 3. deel de 56. en FORESTUS in zyn 21. B. de 26ste: waarn: verdeeling 3. hebben aangeteekend.

Ja zelf *het hert is niet vry van wurmen*, zie hier van de 13de: aanm: der duytſchen op het 9. en 10de. Jaar.

Dat'er *wurmen in de aderen* zyn, beſchrijft JO: RHODIUS; de 6ste: aanm: hebbende de zelve ook in de lieſchtakken ontdekt, zie de 61ste: aanm:

PETRUS BORELLUS, verteld van dierkens de welke de gedaante van een walviſch hebbende, in het bloed zich onthouden. Zie zyn 4de: waarn: in de 3de: verdeeling.

FORETUS wil, dat de koortſzige menſchen met wurmen bezet zyn, zie zyn 7. B. de 36ste: waarn: het eerſte deel.

KIRCHERUS, ſtelt hen als oorzaaken, of werktuygen van de peſtziekte.

RHODIUS, maakt gewag van *een overmaatige, groote wurm* en noemt hem de *oorzaak van eene langduurige ziekte en den dood*, in zyn 3de: deel de 64ste: waarn.

Waar

Waar HILDANUS en andere *wurmen* vonden, gelyk *in de galblaas*, *pisblaas* en elders, is vooren gezegt: maar de H: duytsche vertoonen hen in de *nieren*, zie op het 3de: Jaar de 405. aanmerk:

Gelyk meest alle aanteekenaars van de voorvallen der ziektens, werk maaken, omtrent de pis hunne waarneemingen te berde te brengen, zoo zyn'er te veel om hen alle te noemen, die *wurmen* in de zelve gevonden hebben. Van hen alle zy dan genoech, te noemen de H: duytsche op het 3. en 4de: Jaar, aanm: 156. het 3. J: waarn: 77. het 6. J: waarn: 31. PECHLINUS 2de: B. waarn: 18. de Deenen in hun 5de: stuk, waarn: 21. BONETUS in zyn voorgem: B. waarn: 33. TULP 2de: B. 43ste: Hoofdst: zie ook de hoogduytsche op het woord *Termites.*

Van *wurmachtig bloed*, met den pis geloost, meld BONETUS in zyn 34ste: aanm. de 29ste: verdeeling van het 3de: Boek, als ook van *een diertje*, *van gedaante als een gulletie*, *leevende met de pis uytgewurpen*, in de 35ste: aanmerk: noch van *een wurm door een zoogende vrouw ter blaaze uytgedreeven*, in de 33ste: waarn:

De *wurmen* onthouden zich ook *in den lyfmoeder*, zie hier van de 7de: aanmerk: op het 9de: en 10de: en de 24ste: op het 8ste: Jaar, verdeeling 2. in des zelfs *scheede* vindze FORESTUS; het 21. B. aanm: 37. in de nader aanteekeningen.

Van *wurmen in de beenen*, *den balzak*; van *een gezwel en blaasken vol wurmen*, melden de hoogduytsche aanteekenaars op het 3de: en vierde Jaar, de 173. waarn: ook op het 7de: Jaar, de 16de: waarn.

In schurft en de pokjens beschryftze BORELLUS, waarn. 72.

In

In puysten, pokjens en den geheelen stand des licchaams, RHODIUS, waarn. 64. verd. 3.

Van *een geheel wurmachtig man* (och! was dit gebrek wat zeldzaam!) maaken de Deenen een aanteekening in hun 3[de]: stuk; waarn. 11.

Zwaare toevallen van *myten*, toond HILDANUS, aanmer. 96. gelyk BONETUS in zyn laatste, verd. 35. een *geduurige voortbrenging van wurmen van kindsbeen, tot eene hooge ouderdom. Van verouderde, verscheidene van gedaante, groote, kleene wurmen en van andere dieren*, zyn alom in alle deelen des licchaams aanteekeningen te vinden: zoo dan, zal nu het geschil, of liever de reedenkaaveling moeten zyn, of deeze dieren, die men toestaat, in de deelen der leevende menschelyke licchaamen, gevonden te werden, oorzaaken van ziektens en hunne bygaande gevolgen kunnen zyn, of niet en wel te meerder, om dat onder andere TH. KERKRING, een man, die in de ontleed-en geneeskunde eenen grooten naam verkreegen heeft, het zelve in twyfel trekt: wanneer zyn Ed: op het 177ste: blad, in de 93ste: zynner aanmerkingen, de onzeekerheid des oordeels, het welk men van de dingen, door en by behulp van vergrootglàzen, in de ontleedkunst, veld, poogt te toonen: leydende deeze onzeekerheid af; 1. uyt de kleenheid van het middepunt deezes gezichts; 2. uyt het veranderen der verwe; 3. uyt het beurtelings bezichtigen eenes zelvigen deels, dat, naamelyken, het geene nu gescheiden lykt, waarelyken vereenigd; ja eèn en licchaamelyken te zaamen gevoegd is:

is: maar naa zeeker vergrootglas en des zelfs maaker: B. Spinosa zeer gepreezen te hebben, voegd hy'er deeze woorden by: *door behulp van welk myn verwonderlyk werktuyg, ik zeer verwonderlyken gezien heb, dat, naamelyken, de darmen, de lever en al het weezen der andere ingewanden, met een oneyndig getal van zeer kleene diertjens gevuld zyn: dan iemand die overweegd, dat een huys, het welk bewoond werd, ſchoon en helder is, maar nochthans door de geduurige onderhouding van de geene die het zelve bewoonen, verſlyt, zal mogen twyfelen, of deeze dierkens, door hunne geduurige beweeging, de zelve bederven, of onderhouwen?*

Schoon my niet onbekend is, welke eene groote ingang, geloof en vertrouwen, niet alleen by het gemeene volk, maar lyder! ook by zommige aanzienelyke perzoonen, de ongegronde naamen van ervaarenheid, voorbeeld en verhaal van zoo genoemde gebeurde zaaken en wat des meerder zy, bekomen en behouden hebben, zal ik echter nu geen ſchrijvers tegengaan, noch aanhaalen, die ziektens en hunne oorzaaken van wurmen en andere dieren in 's menſchen licchaam ontkennen, of afleyden: want, om zoo vryhertig, als eerbiediglyken, myn meening te zeggen; ik meen, dat alle ervaaring, aanmerking en voorbeeld, nooit, of maar eenigzints in het algemeen, toch nooit in het bizonder, te paſſe komt.

Eerſtelyken, men ziet nooit twee gevallen, wat zeg ik gevallen, men ziet nooit twee dingen, alom eveneens. Op dien ſtelregel zeide ik eens en het behaagde zommige,

ELK DING IS GODDELYK, OM 'T EEUWIG ONDERSCHEID.

Men passe dit op de geneezkunst toe en voor myn gedachten zullen de tyd des Jaars, tyd des leevens, kunne der lyders, wyze van leeven, plaats der gebreeken, zwaarder, of minder kragt der ziekte en des gebreks; voorts noch veele andere omstandigheden, tegen de evenreedenheid en toepasselykheid van eene aanmerking, op een ander voorval, pleiten.

Ten 2den: vind men weinig menschen en noch minder geneezheeren en heelmeesters, die hunne misslagen, ten nutte van hunne evennaasten, willen, of durven bekennen.

Ten 3den: het gebeurde nu, dat men nâa reedelyk onderzoek, twee zeer naar overeenkomende gevallen aantrof: zoo vraage ik (my dunkt met reeden) besluyt men daar reedelyken een onwederspreekelyke waarheid en gevolgelyke wet, van altyd gebeuren en van altyd als eerst te moeten doen, uyt? Ik meene neen. Men doe hier by, dat:

Ten 4den: geen mensch in de geneez- en heelkunst moet, noch mag aangaan op getuygen; ging dit door en was alles waar, daar men getuygen toe kon vinden, zoo waaren eerlang al de wonderwerken, welke ooit de Pausgezinden ter versiering van hun kraam uytdochten, waar gemaakt: ging dit door, zoo zou men op de getuygenis en verzeekering van een verschrikt, of onkundig mensch duyzend zotternyen, voor waare zaaken, moeten aanneemen en quakzalvers

zalvers den prijs, boven wijze geneezheeren en verſtandige heelmeeſters, behaalen.

Ten 5den: Wat geloof is 'er toch veel aan het verhaal van zaaken te ſlaan, by welken de menſchen, naar zy de zelve verhaalen, nut, of ſchaade behaalen. Wat doed meenig menſch en zeeker wat meenig geneezheer om voordeel niet? te zeggen (toch met een te liegen) *ik heb deeze van doofheid, met dit inſtrument, die van de vallende ziekte, met dat medicament, geneezen*, gaat wel; tot dat men die geneezene luyden zoekt en al heel niet, of wel het tegendeel in hen bevind. Kortom ik houde my aan de regelmaat van reeden, de zelve, zoo veel ik kan, gebruykende, my van mynne uyterlijke zinnen en der zelver hulpmiddelen dienende, gelijk van een bode, tot een brief, een werktuyg, tot het werk, het licht, tot zichtbaar onderſcheid, der in zich reeds onderſcheidene dingen en zoo voorts: vaſtſtellende dat alle ziektens (ik zwyge van uytwendiglijken toegebragte ſchaade) in de vloedige deelen eerſt, ten 2den: in de buyzen, waar door de zelve vloeyen en ten 3den: in de deelen, waar in de zelve werden gevoerd, te vinden zyn: dat wyders, meerdermaalen dan men denkt, dieren, oorzaak van deezer drien deelen quaade geſteltheid, hindernis in beweeging en der zelver gevolgen zyn; ontkennende wel uytdrukkeljjken, dat het bloed en de gal gemaakt, of ooit geſteld zyn, gelijkerwys hen veele beſchryven. Gemeenelijken hebben het deeze deelen en ſtoffen gedaan, gemeenelijken werden zy en hun quaade geſteltenis, de oorzaaken van ziektens genoemt. Het eerſte

 is 'er

is 'er te veel, of te weinig; nu te zout, dan te lymachtig; nu te wrangzuur, dan te waterachtig, nu te dik, dan te dun. Het tweede te veel, of te weinig; te taay, of niet taay genoech; te bitter, of niet bitter naar behooren, nu te naauw, dan niet naauw genoech met het bloed verbonden en vermengt; nu aangebrand, dan niet genoech gekookt. Al deeze praat kan door den beugel en waarom niet? de *visite* krygt 'er zyn beslag, zyn *forma* en de quakzalvende *visitateur* zyn geld door. Die het afbeeldzel van zoo

EEN RAADSHEER MET EEN P, IN 'T MIDDEN, OF VOOR AAN,

by letterschildery; wil zien, leeze de 7[de]: zeedeprint van den Heere van ZUYLICHEM: maar menge onder dien hoop, geen braave en geleerde mannen, die het spoor van reeden en betaamen houdende, God en menschen, om hunne wijsheid en dienst van eere, aan hunne lydende evennaasten, ter goeder trouwe besteed, aangenaam zyn. De zulke weeten uyt de gedaante, het maakzel, de beweeging, dat het bloed niet zout, niet zuur, de gal niet aangebrand, niet waterachtig kan zyn; dat de by-en toemenging van andere, geen deel van weezen, of in zich veranderd: de zulke zoeken geen oorzaaken van ziektens in vochten en werktuygen, die ter plaatze, daar men het begin van de ziekte steld, niet zyn, of ooit waaren: de zulke zullen kunnen en willen begrijpen, dat diertjens, al zien zy de zelve by geen duyzenden en juyst vaademen en voeten lang en dik,

noch

noch altijd ten neuze en ooren van de lijders en lijken uytkruypen, den menſch, in welke zy zyn, ziektens en ſchaaden kunnen toebrengen: ja wel toeſtaan, wijl men in alle deelen des licchaams dieren kan vinden, dat zy ook in alle deelen des licchaams ongemakken kunnen veroorzaaken en waarſchynnelijken veroorzaaken.

Ik vonde ooit en altijd, meerder werk in het onderzoeken en kennen der ziektens en hunne oorzaaken, dan om de zelve, gevonden hebbende, te geneezen, of te hulpe te komen: ja zie de zaaken, welke men meermaalen als oorzaaken van iets ſteld, voor der zelver gevolgen en uytwerkzelen aan. Zoo noemt men een watergezwel in den buyk, een zweer in de long, of lever, een buyl in de lieſch en zoo voorts, wanneer men de zelve in de lijken vind, de oorzaaken van de ziekte en den dood; zonder te denken, dat de zelve de gevolgen van vooraf gebrookene, verſlopte, of anderzints beſchaadigde pijpen en verhinderde beweegingen eeniger vochten zyn; zonder te onderzoeken waar door, in welke plaats, wanneer, op wat wyze deeze zyn geſchied, of hebben kunnen geſchieden. Hier door komt het, dat men, tot een en zelve gebrek, den een geneez-middelen vol vluchtig zout, den ander, welker zaamenſtel aarachtig en vaſt is, ziet gebruyken: maar hier van breeder, by andere gelegenheid, om niet te wijd van mynne ſchrijfſtof te gaan. Ik heb, immers zoo ik meen, genoech getoond, hoe zommige diertjens in de licchaamen der menſchen komen; de wijze nu, op welke zy de zelve kunnen beſchaadigen, pijnigen,

ver-

verwoesten en aldus oorzaaken van ziektens en hunne toevallen ; ja den dood zyn ; verbeelde ik my te zyn , dat deeze dieren , welker duyzende zomtijds by een gevonden werden ,

Eerstelijken de deelen , waar in zy huysvesten , boven maaten uytspannen , zoo door den aanwas van hunne licchaamtjens , als door de vermeerdering van hun geslacht.

2den: Met in en door deeze deelen te bijten , aldus de zelve te verbreeeken , verliezende daar door die werktuygen hun gebruyk in het geheel , of ten deelen.

3den: Met in en door pijpen en plaatzen te booren en zich te wringen , wier tedere zaamenstel hier door in lyen geraakt.

4den: Door broeying der zappen , als zy , naamelijken , den voort-en uytgang der zelve beletten en hinderlijk zyn.

5den: Met de vochten , zappen en stoffen , welke ten voedzel en wasdom , of bereiding en ten dienste van zommige deelen geschikt zyn , tot hun voedzel en wasdom naar zich neemen.

6den: Met hunne vuylicheden , eyeren , jongen , versturvene licchaamtjens tusschen en in de deelen te werpen , wier beweeging aldus verhinderd zynde , quaade gevolgen met zich sleept.

Hier-waaren meerder wijzen van beschaadigen by te doen , maar ik vertrouwe dat deeze genoech zullen zyn , om een denkbeeld van noch andere te maaken.

Die nu een middel weet en gebruykt , het welk , zonder leed aan de deelen des licchaams te doen , deeze

dieren,

dieren, hunne knaaging, kruyping en wat des meerder boven genoemd is, dood, voorkomt, of wel de zelve leevende ten lyve uytwerpt, gaat, ten deezen opzichte, in zyn voorschrift en geneezing zeeker: maar men stonde nu al toe, dat de ongeregeldheden der vloeybaare deelen en alzoo die van het bloed en daar bygemengde stoffen, het zy de wanorder in der zelver gesteldheid, of beweeging gesteld werde, oorzaaken van zommige ziektens en hunne gevolgen kunnen zyn, zal daarom onreedelyk genoemd werden? te willen bewyzen, dat ook dieren in de zelve gemengt; ja in de vaste deelen gevonden werdende, oorzaaken van zommige ziektens en hunne gevolgen kunnen zyn: van het eerste kan men meerder woorden, van het twede daadelyker bewyzen voorbrengen, derhalven was het wel betaamelyk, dat de menschen, die alom en alleenelyken op hunne ervaaringen steunen, door het twede, naar het geene zy wel eerst behoorden te zoeken, te weeten, de reeden, zich geliefden te laaten leyden.

Ik zou wyder nu van de bovengeeyschte geneezmiddelen in het algemeen en bizonder spreeken, vreesde ik niet alreeds de wet van bescheidenheid, het opschrift van deeze verhandeling en de bepaaling van een geschrift, alleen tot eèn oogwit geschikt, overtreden te hebben: houdende, naamelyken, UE: te lang van zyn bezigheden en met zaaken op, welke eygentlyken tot zynne oefening niet behooren: rekkende de redenering langer, dan wel de naam van een brief vereyscht en in de zelve andere zaaken, by mynne ervaaringen, omtrent deeze diert-

E jens

jens genoomen, voegende; maar dit alle zal UE: en elk, die ooit de moeite mag neemen van dit geschrift te leezen, wel kunnen ten besten duyen, wanneer hy in zal zien, dat ik dit alleen ten nutte van de geneezkunde en ten spoore van yverige onderzoekers der noch verborgene kennisse veeler zaaken, welker getal voorwaar onbepaald is, gedaan heb; zullende ook, ter eerster gelegenheid, UE: mynne gedachten, aangaande de buyzen, de Trompetten van FALLOPIUS genoemd en andere daar omtrent gelegene deelen, over welke UE: my de eere doed van te schrijven, gedienstelyken voordragen.

Leyden den 21sten: Maart.
in het Jaar 1698.

COLOPHON

This is volume XVIII of the series

DUTCH CLASSICS IN HISTORY OF SCIENCE

which is published under the supervision of the Netherlands Society for the History of Medicine, Mathematics and Exact Sciences.

The facsimile of the Brief van G. Bidloo aan Antony van Leeuwenhoek (Delft, 1698) was made after the copy in the Library of the Faculty of Veterinary Sciences at the University of Utrecht, with kind permission of the librarian.
The original of the portrait, which represents Bidloo in the year 1710, is a painting by J. F. de la Court, preserved in the Municipal Museum „De Lakenhal", Leyden.
The introduction and the translation, both written by Dr. J. Jansen, were translated into English by Miss C. Dikshoorn.
Printing of introduction and translation: N.V. Drukkerij Trio, The Hague.
Printing of the facsimile: Nederlandsch Drukkerij Bedrijf N.V., Leyden.

The present edition – *limited to fivehundred copies* – is published by

B. DE GRAAF * NIEUWKOOP * NETHERLANDS